T0348443

Diversity, Equity, and Inclusion in Veterinary Medicine, Part II

Editor

CHRISTINA V. TRAN

VETERINARY CLINICS OF NORTH AMERICA: SMALL ANIMAL PRACTICE

www.vetsmall.theclinics.com

November 2024 • Volume 54 • Number 6

ELSEVIER

1600 John F. Kennedy Boulevard • Suite 1800 • Philadelphia, Pennsylvania, 19103-2899

http://www.vetsmall.theclinics.com

**VETERINARY CLINICS OF NORTH AMERICA: SMALL ANIMAL PRACTICE Volume 54, Number 6
November 2024 ISSN 0195-5616, ISBN-13: 978-0-443-31328-8**

Editor: Stacy Eastman

Developmental Editor: Varun Gopal

Veterinary Clinics of North America: Small Animal Practice (ISSN 0195-5616) is published bimonthly by Elsevier Inc., 360
Park Avenue South, New York, NY 10010-1710. Months of issue are January, March, May, July, September, and
November. Business and Editorial Offices: 1600 John F. Kennedy Blvd., Ste. 1800, Philadelphia, PA 19103-2899.
Customer Service Office: 3251 Riverport Lane, Maryland Heights, MO 63043. Periodicals postage paid at New York,
NY and additional mailing offices. Subscription prices are $391.00 per year (domestic individuals), $100.00 per year (domestic students/residents), $503.00 per year (Canadian individuals), $544.00 per year (international individuals), $100.00
per year (Canadian students/residents), and $220.00 per year (international students/residents). For institutional access
pricing please contact Customer Service via the contact information below. To receive student/resident rate, orders must
be accompanied by name of affiliated institution, date of term, and the *signature* of program/residency coordinator on
institution letterhead. Orders will be billed at individual rate until proof of status is received. Foreign air speed delivery is
included in all *Clinics* subscription prices. All prices are subject to change without notice. Orders, claims, and journal inquiries: Please visit our Support Hub page https://service.elsevier.com for assistance.

Reprints. For copies of 100 or more of articles in this publication, please contact the Commercial Reprints Department,
Elsevier Inc., 360 Park Avenue South, New York, NY 10010-1710. Tel.: 212-633-3874; Fax: 212-633-3820; E-mail:
reprints@elsevier.com.

Veterinary Clinics of North America: Small Animal Practice is also published in Japanese by Inter Zoo Publishing Co.,
Ltd., Aoyama Crystal-Bldg 5F, 3-5-12 Kitaaoyama, Minato-ku, Tokyo 107-0061, Japan.

Veterinary Clinics of North America: Small Animal Practice is covered in *Current Contents/Agriculture, Biology and Environmental Sciences, Science Citation Index, ASCA, MEDLINE/PubMed (Index Medicus), Excerpta Medica, and BIOSIS.*

Contributors

EDITOR

CHRISTINA V. TRAN, DVM
Dean, School of Veterinary Medicine, Hanover College, Hanover, Indiana, USA; Multicultural Veterinary Medical Association, Silverdale, Washington, USA

AUTHORS

ANGIE ARORA, MSW, RSW
Veterinary Social Worker & Founder of Arora Wellness, Ontario, Canada

MICHAEL BLACKWELL, DVM, MPH
Director, Program for Pet Health Equity, The University of Tennessee, Knoxville, Tennessee, USA

STEPHEN NIÑO CITAL, RVT, SRA, RLAT, CVPP, VTS-LAM
Lab Manager, Department of Neurobiology, HHMI at Stanford University, Stanford, California, USA; Chief Veterinary Nursing Officer, Remedy Veterinary Specialists, San Francisco, California, USA

KATHERINE FOGELBERG, DVM, PhD (Science Education)
Regional Doctor Mentor, Thrive Pet Healthcare, Austin, Texas, USA

EMILIA WONG GORDON, DVM
Diplomate American Board of Veterinary Practitioners (Shelter Medicine Practice); Veterinary Consultant, Haven Veterinary Services, Vancouver, British Columbia, Canada

SOHAILA JAFARIAN, DVM, MPH
Board Member for the Multicultural Veterinary Medical Association, Board Member for Animal Humane New Mexico, Relief Veterinarian for Jafarian Relief Services, LLC, Albuquerque, New Mexico, USA

CORETTA PATTERSON, DVM
Diplomate, American College of Veterinary Internal Medicine–Small Animals; PG Cert Vet Med Ed, Dean, Midwestern University College of Veterinary Medicine, Downers Grove, Illinois, USA

MONICA DIXON PERRY, BS, CVPM
Director of Veterinary Consulting Services, Burzenski & Co, PC, East Haven, Connecticut, USA

MARIE SATO QUICKSALL, DVM, CVA
Treasurer and Founding Board Member, Multicultural Veterinary Medical Association, Silverdale, Washington, USA

MONAE ROBERTS, MEd, MA
Chief Diversity Officer, UC Davis School of Veterinary Medicine, Davis, California, USA

ISSA ROBSON, BSc Animal Physiology, BVM&S, MRCVS, MSc Ruminant Nutrition
Lecturer in Farm Veterinary Clinical Practice, Department of Veterinary Clinical Science, University of Surrey, Guildford, United Kingdom; Co-Founder, British Veterinary Ethnicity & Diversity Society, Director of Affinity Futures Consultancy Ltd

CAMIA TONGE, MS, LVT, VTS (SAIM)
Clinical Educator, Schwarzman Animal Medical Center, New York, New York, USA

Contents

Pause for a moment to visualize a scenario tinged with somber reflection rather than celebration. Consider the life of an elderly woman, a retired public servant whose career as a librarian enriched countless individuals in her community. Now, in the tranquil latter years of her life, she faces a formidable challenge. Her cherished cat, a steadfast companion throughout her serene retirement, has fallen severely ill. The exorbitant cost of necessary medical treatment cast a long, dark shadow over their future together, ultimately leading to the heart-wrenching decision to euthanize, as the financial burden posed an insurmountable barrier to recovery.

Veterinary medicine is one of the least diverse professions in terms of race and ethnicity. Inclusive mentorship has the potential to increase representation and retention of BIPOC (black, indigenous, people of color) individuals and individuals with other marginalized identities in the field. Inclusive mentorship benefits not only the mentors and mentees but also the veterinary profession and the communities we serve. It is critical to incorporate inclusion principles throughout the mentoring relationship, starting with creating an inclusive environment and considering inclusion in program design and mentor training. Inclusion is an ongoing process that requires dedication and maintenance.

Angie Arora

Veterinary medicine has embarked on a journey of understanding the factors impacting the psychological, emotional, physical, and social health of its people. Discussions of diversity, equity, inclusion, and belonging must address wellbeing; discussions of wellbeing must address diversity, equity, inclusion, and belonging. The profession and the world at large have failed to draw a direct correlation between the two. This article sheds light onto the inextricable link between the two so that no one is left behind as the health of the profession and its people advances.

Sohaila Jafarian

This article examines how culturally responsive care can enhance veterinary medicine by focusing on the interpersonal relationships between veterinarians, their teams, and pet owners. It begins by exploring the historical context of trust within veterinary practice and addresses stereotypes in pet ownership demographics, reinforcing the universal human-animal bond. The article outlines the components of culturally responsive care, noting the scarcity of research in veterinary settings and drawing extensively on the substantial research from human medicine, particularly nursing. It redefines veterinarians as trusted caregivers and details the benefits of culturally responsive care, advocating for more inclusive practices to inspire a more empathetic and culturally competent veterinary community.

Issa Robson

For those new to the concept of allyship, this article will outline some of the foundation skills of allyship and strategies to overcome common hurdles. For those who consider themselves further along their allyship journey, there is material to encourage more effective or strategic allyship activities. Readers are encouraged to reflect on the different ways they can practice allyship within their own organizations. For leadership and management, we outline why allyship is important in veterinary workplaces and set out some key organization changes that can build inclusive workplaces through allyship.

Monae Roberts

It is a well-known fact in veterinary medicine that the field has struggled to diversify the profession and is one of the most homogenous careers in the United States. Discrimination is still quite common in the United States, despite decades of policy changes and implementation of DEI practices. This study discusses how veterinary medicine can benefit from an intersectional approach to diversity, equity, and inclusion. It discusses the need of intersectional data to better understand the disparities that exist within veterinary medicine to make a more significant impact.

The concept of equity recognizes historical and current barriers and promotes thriving for veterinary teams and people and animals in the community. Veterinary medicine lacks sociodemographic diversity; veterinarians and other team members who identify with systemically excluded groups offer valuable contributions but are at risk of workplace discrimination. Client families who face barriers for financial and other reasons are at risk of poor animal health and welfare outcomes, including separation from their animals. This article is part one of 2 articles reviewing how the concept of equity applies and could transform well-being in companion animal veterinary practice in North America.

The concept of equity recognizes historical and current barriers and promotes thriving for veterinary teams and people and animals in the community. It is possible to design equitable workplace systems to prevent and respond to harm using learnings from human medicine and the social sciences. These systems are grounded in the principles of health equity and must incorporate both formal policies and intentional cultivation of supportive culture and relationships. This article is part 2 of 2 articles reviewing how the concept of equity applies and could transform well-being in companion animal veterinary practice in North America.

Teams composed of racially diverse individuals from varied backgrounds offer broader experiences, insights, and methods in clinical approaches, communication, and may offer cultural familiarity to clients. Prioritizing diversity, equity, inclusion, and belonging on ethical grounds is essential, but the advantages of engaging Black, Indigenous, and other People of Color (BIPOC) individuals in clinical specialist roles surpass ethical considerations alone. Research and industry data show a clear link between team diversity and better patient outcomes and business performance, notably in profitability and market expansion. How to engage BIPOC individuals in pursuing veterinary technician specialization, along with its challenges are multifaceted but achievable.

VETERINARY CLINICS OF NORTH AMERICA: SMALL ANIMAL PRACTICE

SERIES OF RELATED INTEREST

Veterinary Clinics: Exotic Animal Practice
https://www.vetexotic.theclinics.com/
Advances in Small Animal Care
https://www.advancesinsmallanimalcare.com/

THE CLINICS ARE NOW AVAILABLE ONLINE!
Access your subscription at:
www.theclinics.com

Preface

Diversity, Equity, and Inclusion in Veterinary Medicine: Continuing to Forge a Path Forward Together

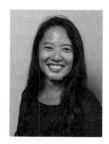

Christina V. Tran, DVM
Editor

In the evolving landscape of veterinary medicine, the importance of diversity, equity, and inclusion (DEI) has never been more evident. As the field expands and adapts to meet the needs of a rapidly diversifying world, it is essential that veterinary professionals not only excel in their clinical competencies but also embrace the principles of DEI to provide compassionate, comprehensive, and culturally responsive care. This publication serves as a guide and a call to action for veterinary professionals to integrate DEI into every facet of their practice, from patient care to professional development and beyond.

One of the most pressing needs in veterinary medicine today is increasing diversity among veterinary professionals, particularly among veterinary technician specialists and boarded veterinary specialists. The profession must reflect the diverse communities it serves to provide care that is both relevant and effective. A diverse workforce brings a range of perspectives, life experiences, and problem-solving approaches that enhance the overall quality of care. It also fosters an environment where innovation thrives, and where clients from all backgrounds feel understood and respected.

Creating an inclusive experience for veterinary clients is another critical component of DEI in veterinary medicine. Inclusivity goes beyond simply welcoming clients from diverse backgrounds; it involves actively and continuously working to understand and meet the unique needs of each client, ensuring that everyone feels heard. A commitment to inclusivity can significantly improve the client experience and, by extension, the health outcomes for their pets.

Access to veterinary care is a fundamental issue that intersects with social equity. Too often, marginalized communities face significant barriers to accessing the care their animals need, whether due to financial constraints, geographic location, or a

Vet Clin Small Anim 54 (2024) ix–x
https://doi.org/10.1016/j.cvsm.2024.08.004
0195-5616/24/© 2024 Published by Elsevier Inc.

lack of culturally responsive care. Addressing these disparities requires a concerted effort to make veterinary care more accessible to all. This publication explores strategies for breaking down these barriers and emphasizes the importance of equity in ensuring that all animals receive the care they deserve, regardless of their owner's background or circumstances.

Inclusive mentorship is essential for nurturing the next generation of veterinary professionals. Mentorship that prioritizes inclusion helps to create a supportive environment where emerging professionals, particularly those from underrepresented groups, can thrive. By providing mentorship that is attuned to the unique challenges faced by diverse individuals, the veterinary field can cultivate a more inclusive and equitable workforce. In addition, it is important to consider the role that allies, advocates, and accomplices play in supporting marginalized veterinary team members.

Supporting the mental health and well-being of a diverse veterinary team is crucial for supporting and sustaining a thriving profession. Veterinary medicine is inherently challenging, and these challenges can be compounded for individuals who face additional stressors related to their marginalized identities. This publication discusses the importance of recognizing and addressing these unique needs, ensuring that all team members have access to the resources and support they need to maintain their well-being.

Culturally responsive care is increasingly recognized as a key component of effective practice. Acknowledging and respecting cultural differences can enhance the relationship between veterinary professionals and their clients, leading to better communication and improved animal health.

Intersectionality in veterinary medicine acknowledges the complex and overlapping identities that individuals bring to the workplace. Recognizing these intersections is crucial for creating an environment where all individuals can thrive. Finally, this publication emphasizes the importance of creating veterinary practices that center equity, something that should be integral to every aspect of veterinary medicine.

As you engage with this publication, I invite you to consider how you can contribute to a more diverse, equitable, and inclusive veterinary profession. Whether through personal actions, institutional changes, or community advocacy, every effort counts in shaping the future of veterinary medicine for the better.

Christina V. Tran, DVM
School of Veterinary Medicine
Hanover College
517 Ball Drive
Hanover, IN, USA

Multicultural Veterinary Medical Association
Silverdale, WA, USA

E-mail address:
tran@hanover.edu

Editorial

Creating an Inclusive Experience for Veterinary Clients

Veterinary medicine is the cornerstone in the lives of countless pet owners. Despite this critically vast and critically important role, the veterinary profession faces significant challenges in diversity, equity, and inclusion (DEI)—both within its professional ranks and in the clientele it serves. As the number of pet-owning households in the United States continues to rise, it becomes more evident that there is an increasing need for veterinary practices to be receptive and supportive of an inclusive environment.

Privately owned veterinary hospitals as well as corporately owned practices, along with their management and leadership teams, are the catalyst to spearheading transformative initiatives that ensure all clients, regardless of their background, feel welcomed, understood, and valued. This article delves into practical strategies for cultivating environments that promote inclusivity, which will be beneficial to both clients and ultimately the veterinary profession.

The following are practical strategies for creating an inclusive environment and enhancing the client experience in veterinary medicine.

TEAM TRAINING IN DIVERSITY, EQUITY, AND INCLUSION

In the increasingly diverse world of veterinary medicine, implementing a robust strategy for DEI is crucial for fostering an inclusive workplace and providing culturally competent care to a diverse client base. A strategic roadmap follows for integrating DEI training within a veterinary hospital, emphasizing the roles of ownership and leadership in ensuring successful implementation.

Establish Clear Diversity, Equity, and Inclusion Goals and Objectives

The *first step* is for the hospital's leadership to clearly define what they aim to achieve with DEI initiatives. This could include enhancing staff cultural competence, improving patient care across diverse populations, and creating an inclusive workplace culture. These goals should be SMART (specific, measurable, achievable, relevant, and time-bound).

The *second step* is assessing your practice's current DEI maturity. Before implementing new training programs, conduct a thorough assessment of the current DEI status within the practice. This might involve surveys, staff interviews, and reviewing patient feedback to identify any existing gaps or areas needing improvement. Understanding the starting point helps tailor the DEI program more effectively to ensure its success.

The *third step* is to develop a comprehensive DEI training program with clear goals and a baseline understanding of the current DEI climate within the veterinary profession while developing a training program tailored to the needs of your individual practice. This program should address various aspects, such as unconscious bias, cultural

Vet Clin Small Anim 54 (2024) xi–xxii
https://doi.org/10.1016/j.cvsm.2024.08.003
0195-5616/24/© 2024 Published by Elsevier Inc.

humility, inclusive communication, and legal aspects of workplace diversity. The training should be interactive, possibly incorporating role-play, workshops, and seminars to engage staff fully.

The *fourth step* is to secure commitment from ownership or executive level management if it is a corporate entity. For DEI initiatives to be successful, they must have full backing from the hospital's ownership and senior leadership. This includes not only verbal endorsement but also active participation in DEI training sessions and public advocacy of the program's importance. Leadership's commitment should be visible and unequivocal, serving as a model for the rest of the team.

The *fifth step* is integrating DEI into organizational policies and practices and revising any existing policies and procedures to reflect the hospital's commitment to diversity and inclusion. This could involve updating hiring practices, patient interaction protocols, and employee evaluation criteria to align with DEI principles. Ensure that these policies are well-documented and accessible to all health care team members.

The *sixth step* is rolling out training to all levels and departments of your health care team. This simply means that across all levels of the organization, from executive management to frontline team members, DEI training should take place. This becomes a part of the practice's onboarding efforts and a clear component of the practice's cultural DNA. It's important to ensure that training is mandatory and tailored to the specific roles and responsibilities of different staff members. Consider ongoing or refresher training sessions to reinforce expected principles and practices.

The *seventh step* includes monitoring, evaluating, and adapting. It is important to continuously monitor the effectiveness of the DEI training by tracking key performance indicators related to workplace diversity, staff satisfaction, and client feedback. Regularly evaluating the impact of the training and making adjustments as needed will set this strategy up for success and demonstrate to your team members and client base the sincere intentions with your efforts as it relates to DEI. This might involve seeking your team's input on their training experience and any changes they feel are needed in the workplace culture as well as interactions with your clients and pet owners.

The *eighth step* is establishing and fostering an open environment for feedback that includes creating mechanisms for your team members to provide anonymous feedback on DEI issues and the training program itself. This could include suggestion boxes, regular team and/or departmental meetings, or dedicated channels for DEI discussions. Encouraging open communication helps identify new issues as they arise and reinforces the importance of transparency and continuous improvement.

The *ninth step* is celebrating diversity and reinforcing DEI values, which includes recognizing and celebrating cultural diversity within the team through events and/or special acknowledgments. Celebrating diversity helps to build a sense of community and belonging while simultaneously reinforcing the value of your practice's DEI initiatives.

The *tenth step* is leveraging external resources by being open to partnerships with DEI experts or organizations that can provide additional resources and perspectives. These partnerships can enhance the training program and provide credibility to the hospital's efforts.

By following these steps, veterinary hospital ownership and leadership can successfully implement a DEI strategy that not only enriches the workplace but also enhances the quality of care provided to diverse communities. This strategic approach ensures that DEI principles are deeply integrated into the fabric of the organization, making them a part of everyday practice rather than a one-time training exercise.

Team training is key and will be foundational to your program's success.

Over and beyond establishing and implementing team training, there are additional steps that should be taken in your practice's strategic approach to creating an inclusive experience for your clients. The aforementioned begins with your health care team and allows them to understand and embrace DEI, making the creation of an inclusive environment for your clients easier.

After establishing and incorporating team training, other key strategies to consider are listed in the remainder of this article.

INCORPORATING MULTILINGUAL SERVICES

Incorporating multilingual services in a veterinary hospital is a pivotal strategy for creating a diverse and inclusive environment, especially in communities with a substantial non–English-speaking population. This approach not only improves communication and trust between the health care team and its clients but also enhances the overall quality of care provided to the pets

Some tips for veterinary hospital ownership and leadership to successfully implement multilingual services follow.

Assessing the Need

The first step in implementing multilingual services is to assess the linguistic needs of the community your veterinary practice serves. This can be achieved by analyzing demographic data, client registration information, and even informal feedback from clients about their language preferences and challenges. Understanding the specific languages spoken by a significant portion of the client base (or potential client base) will help tailor the services to meet community needs effectively.

Hiring Bilingual Staff

Recruiting bilingual team members is perhaps the most straightforward approach to offering multilingual services. When hiring, prioritize candidates who are fluent in the languages most commonly spoken by your client base. It is also important to provide appropriate compensation for those employees that are multilingual. In addition, consider the cultural competence of these employees, as understanding cultural nuances is as important as language skills in providing excellent care and service.

Training

For existing team members who are interested, provide opportunities for language training to enhance their communication skills. Encouraging team members to become trained and educated in medical Spanish, for example, can be particularly useful in areas with a high Hispanic population. This not only improves the inclusiveness of your services but also boosts team engagement and development.

Utilize Technology

Leverage technology to bridge any language gaps. This can include the use of translation apps, bilingual digital kiosks for check-in processes, and Web sites that offer information in multiple languages. Ensure that all electronic communications, such as appointment reminders and follow-up e-mails, are available in the preferred languages of your clients.

Utilize Professional Interpretation Services

In scenarios where bilingual staff are not available, or for less commonly spoken languages, contracting professional interpreters is a vital resource. These services can be scheduled for appointments or can be accessed on-demand via phone or video calls. It is essential to use interpreters who are familiar with medical terminology to ensure accurate and efficient communication.

Cultural Humility Training

Provide regular training on cultural humility to all staff, not just those who speak multiple languages. Understanding cultural differences in pet ownership practices, communication styles, and decision-making processes is crucial for delivering respectful, effective, and culturally responsive care.

Feedback Mechanisms

Implement systems to gather feedback specifically about the effectiveness and accessibility of multilingual services. This could include surveys, focus groups, or suggestion boxes, which should also be available in multiple languages. Use this feedback to continually improve language services.

Community Engagement

Actively engage with local communities through educational programs, participation in cultural events, and partnerships with community organizations. This not only raises awareness about your services but also builds trust within the community.

Visibility of Multilingual Services

Make it known that your veterinary practice offers multilingual services. This includes signage in multiple languages within the hospital, as well as multilingual marketing materials. Visibility is key to ensuring that all potential clients are aware that these services are available.

Regular Review and Adaptation

Finally, regularly review the effectiveness of your multilingual services. This includes analyzing utilization rates, client satisfaction, and financial impacts. Be prepared to adapt your strategy as the community's needs change or as you gather more insights from your ongoing efforts. By implementing these steps, veterinary hospitals can ensure that their services are accessible to a diverse client base, thereby not only enhancing client satisfaction and loyalty but also promoting better health outcomes for the pets they serve.

ESTABLISH CULTURAL SENSITIVITY

Implementing cultural sensitivity in a veterinary practice is crucial for creating a diverse and inclusive environment that respects and understands the varied cultural backgrounds of its clients.

Practical tips follow for integrating cultural sensitivity into the everyday operations your veterinary practice.

Incorporating Diverse Hiring Practices

Actively seek to hire staff from diverse backgrounds. A team that reflects the community's demographic diversity can provide better insights into the cultural needs of your clients and offer a more comfortable environment for a multicultural clientele. This diversity will also provide a deeper understanding and empathy within the team.

Implement Client-Centered Communication

Ensure that communication styles are adapted to meet the diverse needs of your clientele. This involves not only language but also understanding the nuances of nonverbal communication, such as eye contact, gestures, and personal space, which can vary significantly between cultures. Train staff to ask open-ended questions that allow clients to express their concerns and preferences regarding their pets' care.

Include Resource Development

Develop resources that cater to the diverse needs of your clients. This could include informational brochures in multiple languages, visual aids that do not rely heavily on text, and instructional videos that depict a variety of cultural groups and include closed captioning. Ensure that these resources are accessible both in the practice and online to reach a broader audience.

Provide Flexible Policies

Adapt your practice policies to be culturally sensitive and flexible to accommodate various cultural practices. For instance, consider how you schedule appointments and manage visits in a way that respects cultural and religious holidays and/or observances.

Institute Community Engagement

Engage with the local community to understand better and serve the cultural needs specific to your area. Participate in community events, host educational events at your practice on topics related to pet care, and invite feedback on how your practice can improve its services. Building relationships with community leaders and groups can also enhance trust and communication.

Provide Feedback Mechanism

Create mechanisms for clients to provide feedback specifically about cultural sensitivity issues. This feedback should be actively reviewed and used to continually refine practices and training. Make it easy and safe for clients to express concerns about cultural insensitivity or miscommunications.

Celebrate Diversity

Embrace and celebrate cultural diversity within your practice. This could include decorating the clinic with culturally diverse themes, celebrating a variety of cultural holidays, or featuring pets and owners from different backgrounds in your marketing materials. By including these principles into the fabric of your veterinary practice, you can build a truly inclusive environment that respects and honors the cultural diversity of your clientele. This commitment not only enhances client satisfaction but also enriches the workplace culture, promoting a deeper understanding and respect among staff and clients alike. You can have your health care team members actively involved in celebrating diversity by tapping into their own diverse cultures and experiences.

PROVIDE AN ACCESSIBLE FACILITY

In order to foster a diverse and inclusive experience, it is fundamental to provide a facility that is accessible and meets the needs of your client base. Practical tips follow for ensuring that your veterinary practice is welcoming and accessible to all clients, regardless of their physical abilities or other needs.

Make Physical Accessibility Improvements

Begin by ensuring that the physical layout of your clinic complies with the Americans with Disabilities Act standards. This includes providing wheelchair-accessible entrances and exits, adequate hallway widths, accessible examination rooms, and restroom facilities. Consider the placement of furniture and the height of counters to ensure they are accessible to everyone, including those in wheelchairs or with mobility impairments.

Provide Clear Signage

Use clear, visible signage throughout the facility. Signs should be easy to read with large fonts and high contrast for those with visual impairments. Include Braille on signage wherever possible. Ensure that directional signs are placed at key points to guide clients through the facility easily.

Become Sensitive to Sensory Needs

Recognize that some clients may have sensory sensitivities. Provide a quiet waiting area away from the main reception to accommodate those who might be overwhelmed by noise. Consider the clinic's lighting—soft, natural lighting is often less distressing than harsh fluorescent lights.

Include Service Animal Awareness Training

Ensure that your team is trained on the proper etiquette and legal requirements regarding service animals. Your health care team should know how to interact with service animals and their owners and recognize that these animals are not pets but working animals with specific roles.

Provide Disability Team Training

Conduct regular training sessions with your team to educate them about various disabilities and how to assist clients with special needs. Training should cover how to offer assistance without being patronizing, the proper use of inclusive language, and understanding the diverse needs of clients with disabilities.

Offer Inclusive Communication Tools

Provide communication tools to assist clients with different needs. This might include having written materials available in large print, offering information in easy-to-understand and pictorial formats, and using technology such as tablets that can display information visually for those who are deaf or hard of hearing.

Establish Emergency Preparedness

Ensure that emergency evacuation procedures include provisions for clients with disabilities. Your team should be trained to assist in evacuations and know how to effectively handle situations involving clients with mobility issues or other impairments.

Provide Flexible Accommodations

Be flexible in your appointment scheduling and procedures to accommodate clients with special needs. For example, allow for longer appointment times for clients who may need additional time for moving between different areas of the clinic or understanding and completing procedures. This not only extends to clients with disabilities but also is applicable with elderly clients.

By implementing these tips, your veterinary practice will not only meet the legal requirements for accessibility but also demonstrate a commitment to inclusivity and respect for all clients, creating a welcoming, inclusive environment that enhances the care and service provided to the community.

INSTITUTE INCLUSIVE MARKETING

Inclusive marketing is essential for veterinary practices aiming to create a welcoming environment that reflects the diversity of their client base. It involves crafting messages that resonate across different backgrounds, abilities, and perspectives, ensuring that all clients feel valued and understood.

Practical tips and examples follow to help veterinary clinics implement effective inclusive marketing strategies.

Include Diverse Representation in Visual Content

Ensure that the imagery used in marketing materials reflects the diversity of your client base and the community. This includes using photos and videos featuring people of various races, ethnicities, ages, genders, and abilities. For example, if creating a brochure or a social media campaign, include images of diverse families with their pets, showing a range of activities and interactions that resonate with different cultural backgrounds.

Provide Language Accessibility

Make sure that your marketing materials are accessible to people who speak different languages. Offering brochures, flyers, Web site content, and social media posts in the predominant languages spoken in your community can significantly enhance accessibility. In addition, consider the readability of your materials, using clear, jargon-free language that is easy to understand for nonnative speakers and people of all educational backgrounds.

Remember Cultural Sensitivity

Understand and respect cultural nuances that might influence how different communities perceive veterinary care. Tailor your messages to address these nuances; for example, highlight how your practice respects traditional views about animal care or offers services that cater to specific cultural practices (like prayer or meditation areas for clients who may need them during their visit).

Highlight Inclusivity Initiatives

Use your marketing platforms to talk about your inclusivity efforts. Share stories or case studies about how you have successfully addressed diverse needs, such as accommodating service animals for people with disabilities or events you've hosted for diverse community groups. This not only markets your services but also builds trust and credibility.

Encourage Social Media Engagement

Engage with diverse audiences on social media by recognizing cultural holidays, awareness months, and significant days from different cultures. Use these occasions to educate your audience about different cultural practices related to pets and to show your practice's involvement and respect for these traditions.

Provide Feedback Mechanisms

Implement and highlight mechanisms for feedback on your marketing efforts. Encourage clients to share their thoughts on how inclusive they find your marketing materials. This can help you understand what works and what may need adjustment.

Provide Training for Marketing Teams

Ensure that your marketing team is trained in DEI principles. Understanding the importance of inclusive marketing and how to effectively implement it is crucial. Regular training sessions can help keep these principles at the forefront of your team's mind as they create campaigns.

Seek out Partnerships with Diverse Community Groups

Collaborate with diverse community groups to extend your marketing reach and enhance the relevance of your messages. These partnerships can provide valuable insights into the needs and preferences of different groups.

Provide Accessible Advertising Channels

Utilize a mix of traditional and digital media to ensure that your marketing messages reach people with varying access to technology. For example, while social media and online ads are powerful tools, do not overlook community radio stations, local newspapers, and bulletin boards in community centers. By incorporating these strategies into your marketing efforts, a veterinary practice can ensure that it not only reaches a broader audience but also resonates more deeply with clients from all walks of life, which in return will foster an environment of inclusion and respect.

INCORPORATE DIVERSE REPRESENTATION IN DECISION MAKING

Diverse representation in decision making processes is crucial for fostering an inclusive environment in a veterinary practice. This ensures that the perspectives and needs of a varied client base are considered, leading to better service delivery and a more welcoming atmosphere.

Practical tips follow for implementing an inclusive and diverse environment that includes representation in decision making.

Build a Diverse Leadership Team

Start by ensuring that the leadership team reflects the diversity of the community and client base. This includes considering gender, race, ethnicity, age, disability status, and other aspects of diversity when making hiring and promotion decisions. A diverse leadership team brings a variety of perspectives and experiences that can lead to more innovative and inclusive decision making.

Establish a Diversity, Equity, and Inclusion Committee

Create a DEI committee that includes members from different backgrounds and roles within the veterinary practice. This committee should meet regularly to discuss and address DEI issues, ensuring that diverse viewpoints are integrated into the practice's policies and strategies. The DEI committee can also be responsible for monitoring the progress of DEI initiatives and making recommendations for improvement.

Engage Team Members at All Levels

Encourage input from staff at all levels of the organization. Implement regular surveys, suggestion boxes, and open forums where employees can share their ideas and feedback on DEI-related matters. Ensure that there is a transparent process for how this feedback is considered and acted upon, demonstrating that all voices are valued.

Establish Inclusive Hiring Practices

Implement hiring practices that prioritize diversity. This includes using diverse job boards, networking with community organizations, and offering internships or mentorship programs to underrepresented groups. Ensure that your hiring efforts is diverse to mitigate unconscious bias during the selection process.

Provide Training on Unconscious Bias

Institute training for all employees, particularly those involved in hiring and decision making, on unconscious bias and its impact. This helps team members recognize and mitigate their own biases, leading to more equitable decision-making processes.

Create Transparent Decision-Making Processes

Ensure that decision-making processes are transparent and inclusive. Clearly communicate how decisions are made, who is involved, and how input from diverse perspectives is incorporated. This transparency builds trust and shows a commitment to inclusive practices.

Promote from Within Whenever Possible

Identify and nurture talent within your organization from diverse backgrounds. Provide professional development opportunities, mentorship, and career development paths that encourage underrepresented employees to aspire to and achieve leadership roles.

Establish a Client Advisory Taskforce

Create an advisory taskforce that include clients from diverse backgrounds. This committee can provide valuable insights into the needs and preferences of different client groups and help guide the practice's policies and services. Engaging clients in this way ensures that the practice remains responsive to the community it serves.

Regularly Review and Update Policies

Continuously review and update your policies and practices to ensure they are inclusive and equitable. This includes everything from team guidelines/handbook to client service protocols. Involve diverse stakeholders in this review process to ensure that policies reflect a wide range of perspectives.

FOCUS ON COMMUNITY ENGAGEMENT

Community is essential for veterinary practices that aim to create a diverse and inclusive environment. Engaging with the community helps build trust, fosters relationships, and ensures that the clinic's services meet the needs of all community members.

Practical tips follow for ensuring that your veterinary practice effectively engages with its community.

Sponsor or participate in local events, such as pet fairs, cultural festivals, health fairs, and neighborhood gatherings, which should include setting up booths or informational tables where your team members have the opportunity to interact with community members, provide educational materials, and offer free services, such as pet health checks or vaccinations. Ensure representation from diverse team members who can connect with various community groups. Offer multilingual materials and have bilingual team members present to and assist non–English-speaking attendees.

Host Educational Workshops and Seminars

Organize workshops on pet care, nutrition, first aid, and common health issues in different languages relevant to your community and clientele. Collaborate with local schools, colleges and/or universities, community centers, and cultural organizations to host these events. Invite speakers from different cultural backgrounds to share their expertise and perspectives on pet care. Use visual aids and hands-on demonstrations to make the information accessible to all attendees.

Form Partnerships with Local Organizations

Partner with animal shelters, rescue groups, schools, and community organizations to create joint initiatives that benefit the community. This could include developing programs that offer discounted or free services to underserved populations. Work with local shelters to host adoption events and provide postadoption support and education. Collaborate with schools to create pet education programs for children, teaching them about responsible pet ownership and the importance of animal welfare.

Establish a Community Advisory Board

Establish a community advisory board consisting of diverse community members who can provide insights and feedback on your services and outreach efforts. Meet regularly with the advisory board to discuss community needs, cultural considerations, and potential areas for improvement. You can then use the board's feedback to tailor services, marketing strategies, and community engagement efforts to better meet the needs of diverse clients. Recognizing and valuing the contributions of the advisory board members ensures their voices are heard and respected.

Volunteer at Charitable Activities

Engage in volunteer activities, such as providing free veterinary services at local shelters or participating in community clean-up events. You can encourage your team to volunteer their time and skills to support local animal welfare initiatives. This opens up the opportunity to organize charity drives to collect food, toys, and other supplies for pets in need within the community. In addition, publicizing these efforts through your marketing channels to demonstrate your clinic's commitment to the community will validate and demonstrate your efforts.

Incorporate Cultural Celebrations and Awareness Campaigns

Celebrate cultural holidays and awareness months by hosting special events and campaigns that highlight different cultures and their relationship with pets. This would include decorating the practice to reflect cultural celebrations and sharing educational materials about the significance of these holidays and how they relate to pet care. There is also the opportunity to run social media campaigns featuring stories and photos from clients and your team members that celebrate these holidays, which can showcase their pets and traditions.

Ensure Social Media Engagement Is Diversity, Equity, and Inclusion Focused

Use social media platforms to engage with the community by sharing relevant content, responding to comments, and hosting interactive sessions. Posting content that reflects the diversity of your community, such as client testimonials, pet care tips in different languages, and stories that highlight various cultural practices related to pet care. You could host live Q&A sessions with veterinarians and team members to address community questions and concerns in real-time. It is also recommended that you encourage user-generated content by inviting clients to share photos and stories of their pets, creating a sense of community and inclusion.

Feedback and Improvement

Implement a system for collecting and acting on feedback from the community to continuously improve your services and engagement efforts. This could include distributing surveys and feedback forms in multiple languages to gather insights from a diverse range of clients. In addition, hold regular open forums where community members can voice their opinions and suggestions. In the end, using this feedback to make tangible changes to your practice and communicating these changes to the community shows that their input is valued.

Implement Educational Outreach Programs

Develop outreach programs targeting specific community groups, such as schools, senior centers, and immigrant communities. You can then tailor educational programs to address the unique needs and concerns of each group, such as pet care for seniors or pet ownership for first-time pet owners from immigrant backgrounds. Your practice will shine as you provide resources and materials in accessible formats and languages to ensure they are useful and informative for all participants. After taking these steps, you should follow up with participants to offer ongoing support and resources, fostering long-term relationships and trust.

By implementing these strategies, veterinary practices can ensure they are engaging with their communities in a meaningful, inclusive way. This not only enhances the client experience but also builds stronger, more trusting relationships with diverse community members, ultimately contributing to the success and growth of your practice.

SUMMARY

Creating an inclusive environment at a veterinary practice is not merely a goal, but a continuous commitment to fostering a culture of respect, understanding, and accessibility for all clients and team members. An inclusive practice goes beyond offering high-quality veterinary care; it encompasses recognizing and valuing the diversity within the community it serves and ensuring that all individuals feel welcomed, understood, and supported.

The journey toward inclusivity begins with leadership. Ownership and management must champion DEI initiatives, setting the tone for the entire practice. This involves establishing clear DEI policies, providing ongoing training for your team, and embedding inclusive practices into every aspect of the practice's operations. By demonstrating a genuine commitment to inclusivity from the top down, veterinary practices can foster a culture where every team member feels valued and empowered to contribute.

One of the most critical aspects of creating an inclusive environment is ensuring diverse representation in decision making. Including voices from various backgrounds and experiences helps the practice to better understand and meet the needs of its diverse client base. Forming DEI committees, creating advisory boards with community members, and ensuring diversity within leadership roles are practical steps to achieve this.

Transparent and inclusive decision-making processes not only improve service delivery but also build trust and loyalty among clients. Community engagement plays a pivotal role in fostering inclusivity. Veterinary practices must actively participate in and contribute to their local communities. This can be achieved through partnerships with local organizations, participation in community events, and hosting educational workshops. Engaging with the community allows practices to build strong, trust-based relationships and ensures that their services are relevant and accessible to all. By celebrating cultural diversity and recognizing the unique needs of different community groups, practices can create a welcoming environment that resonates with a broad audience.

Implementing multilingual services is another essential component of an inclusive practice. Offering materials and services in multiple languages ensures that non–English-speaking clients receive the same level of care and understanding as their English-speaking counterparts. This not only improves client satisfaction but also broadens the practice's reach within the community.

Creating an accessible facility is fundamental to inclusivity. This means ensuring that the physical environment accommodates people of all abilities and providing clear, easy-to-understand information about services and procedures. By removing physical and communicative barriers, veterinary practices can make their services accessible to everyone.

Finally, inclusive marketing strategies are vital for communicating the practice's commitment to diversity and inclusion. Marketing materials should reflect the diversity of the community and be designed to resonate with different cultural groups. This involves using diverse imagery, multilingual content, and culturally sensitive messaging.

In conclusion, creating an inclusive environment at a veterinary practice is a dynamic, ongoing process that requires dedication, empathy, and proactive engagement. By prioritizing DEI initiatives, involving diverse voices in decision making, engaging with the community, implementing multilingual services, ensuring accessibility, and adopting inclusive marketing strategies to name a few approaches, veterinary practices can create a welcoming and supportive environment for all clients. This will not only enhance client satisfaction and loyalty but also contribute to the overall success of your practice.

Monica Dixon Perry, BS, CVPM
Burzenski & Co, PC
East Haven, CT, USA

E-mail address:
Mdixonperry823@gmail.com

FURTHER READINGS

American Veterinary Medical Association DEI resources. Available at: https://www.avma.org/resources-tools/diversity-and-inclusion-veterinary-medicine. Accessed.
Veterinary Medical Association Executives DEI resources. Available at: https://vmae.org/resources/diversity-and-inclusion/. Accessed.

Editorial

Diversity in Veterinary Specialty Medicine: A Robust History with Scant Documentation

The practical procedure to recant the early history of Tuskegee University School of Veterinary Medicine (USVM) would be to examine the writing and record of the period. Historians oftentimes find a paucity of records that impede their studies. This does not mean that little of importance occurred; rather, it represents that no one took the time to record what was done, or in some instances, valuable historical records were unintentionally destroyed...

TS Williams, 2nd Dean of Tuskegee University School of Veterinary Medicine (USVM)

Diversity encompasses a lot; it can mean different things to different people, and anyone you ask to define it may give you a slightly different answer. *Oxford Languages*, Google's preferred online dictionary, defines diversity as: "the state of being diverse; variety," and "the practice or quality of including or involving people from a range of different social and ethnic backgrounds and of different genders, sexual orientations, etc."[1] But so often when we consider diversity in the field of veterinary medicine or veterinary specialty medicine, people think about primarily gender, then race and ethnicity, hard stop. Which means that so many other forms of diversity are left out: socioeconomic diversity, disability, religious affiliation, LGBTQIA+ status, neurodiversity, immigrant status and so on.

While we cannot take on all forms of diversity in this essay, we do hope to describe some of the advancements in veterinary specialty medicine with regards to race and ethnicity, while also discussing the lack of diversity information in general that has and continues to occur within this very small subset of the veterinary profession. It is wonderful to see racial/ethnic diversity within the specialty fields, but it is also a challenge to find it. And seeing/finding other types of diversity—disability, neurodivergence, LGTBQIA+, religious, and the like—is often even more challenging. It is great that the many previously existing barriers to achieving a veterinary degree and specialty certification are slowly but surely become less and less towering, but visibility across the profession and within the specialty fields continues to be an issue. We do know, however, that representation matters, and that without it, the status quo continues to roll forward.

But how do we know that diversity—of any kind—matters within the profession? It is strongly supported within the human health care fields that patients feel more confident in their care when they have race-concordance. Why? Because people are more likely to seek medical care from someone who looks like them; this affinity provides a level of comfort to patients because they feel less likely to be judged and more likely to be listened to.[2,3] Another important reason for increasing racial/ethnic diversity in human medicine is that physicians who identify as either Black/African American or Hispanic/Latino are far more likely to work in areas where there are higher concentrations of

Vet Clin Small Anim 54 (2024) xxiii–xxx
https://doi.org/10.1016/j.cvsm.2024.08.005
0195-5616/24/© 2024 Published by Elsevier Inc.

underserved minorities of a similar racial/ethnic background.[4,5] And while one comprehensive review of the literature was unable to find a correlation between patient-provider race-concordance and positive health outcomes for underserved patient populations,[6] the literature is supportive that such concordance at least increases the chances that underserved populations will access care and feel better about their care when racial concordance exists. Studies have also documented this issue in Native Americans as well as with Asian Americans.[7,8]

While the veterinary literature is scant to absent in this area of research, it is not unreasonable to make the leap that if this is true of physicians, it is likely to be at least somewhat true in veterinary medicine, too. Thus, in writing about diversity and veterinary specialty medicine, it bears taking time to point out some truths about the profession as a whole. The first veterinary school in the United States was Iowa State University, which offered its first class in veterinary medicine in 1872, though it was not officially founded until 1879.[9] While statistics about its first graduating class could not be found on open-access sites, it is probably safe to say that most—if not all—graduates for the first decades were white men. Looking at the Deans of the program, one can see that all Deans from 1879 to 2011 were white men. From 2011 to 2017, Dean Lisa K. Nolan (white woman) came on board, and since 2018, it has been Dean Dan Grooms, another white man. This is not intended to call out Iowa State by any means; a casual perusal of the Deans of the majority of accredited colleges of veterinary medicine across the United States and Canada reveals a very similar profile. This is supported by the research. In 2020, Gill and Singh[10] reported that veterinary program Deans in the United States and Canada from 1966 to 2018 were 91% white men, 5% white women, and 4% ethnic minorities. And Vezeau and colleagues[11] reported in 2024 that women continue to be underrepresented in leadership within academia worldwide, though they did not examine minority representation within their research.

This is likely not surprising; if we consider the progression of diversity within the profession, it appears to mirror that of diversity within the United States, starting with primarily white men, moving toward including white women, then beginning to see Black men, and finally, encompassing Black women. This leaves out, of course, the emergence of Asian Americans, Latino/Hispanic Americans, Native Americans, and Asian American Pacific Islanders, who are even more difficult to find historical records about within the veterinary profession. In fact, when researching this article, attempts to find the first Asian American, Latinx/Hispanic, and Native American veterinary graduates from US programs were unsuccessful. There is equal lack of information about the first 2SLGBTQIA+ US veterinary graduates and those with disabilities. In fact, the earliest mention of disabled veterinarians one author was able to find is dated 2004,[12] reporting on a study in the United Kingdom about this topic that started in 2000.

Indeed, the individual to earn the first Doctor of Veterinary Medicine degree in the United States was Dr Daniel E. Salmon, as an 1876 graduate of Cornell's veterinary program; he would go on to become the first chief of the Bureau of Animal Industry and was, not surprisingly, a white man.[13] It would not be until 1903 that the first white woman would graduate from a veterinary college—Dr Mignon Nicolson, although Dr Elinor McGrath is often considered to be the first female veterinarian.[14] Dr Florence Kimball would graduate around the same time as Dr McGrath in 1910, from Cornell's College of Veterinary Medicine.[14,15] All three were white women.

The first African American man to graduate from a veterinary school in the United States was Dr Augustus Nathan Lushington, a Black man who earned his degree from the University of Pennsylvania in 1897,[16] although the *Journal of Veterinary Medical Education* reported that Dr Henry Stockton was the first graduate in 1889 from the Harvard School of Veterinary Medicine.[14] The fact that records are not clear about such statistics is a statement in itself. It would not be until 1949 that a Black woman would earn the degree; in fact, two Black female veterinarians joined the profession that year: Dr Alfreda Johnson Webb from Tuskegee and Dr Jane Hinton from the University of Pennsylvania.[17,18]

We could continue providing a timeline of the veterinary profession in the United States, but it should be pretty clear that the majority of veterinarians in the United States have been white since the inception of the profession in the country. There were, of course, barrier breakers—not only those who were not white or male, but also those who were members of other underserved groups that bring such diversity to any profession (eg, disabled, neurodiverse, LGBTQIA+, first-generation scholars, and the like). Unfortunately, it is difficult to find and accurately report diversity information in this profession as a whole; when looking at diversity in the specialty colleges, it becomes even more challenging. And that's just looking at racial and ethnic diversity.

It is important to keep in mind that just because we were not formally documented does not mean that we were not around or were not looking to build the support lacking from the profession as a whole. The first affinity group reported was the Women's Veterinary Association, which met for the first time in 1947 at the Cincinnati American Veterinary Medical Association (AVMA) convention.[19] It was started by Dr Mary Knight Dunlap and continued for 66 years, dissolving in 2014 and being re-created as the Association for Women Veterinarians Foundation in 2005.[19,20] Other affinity groups would follow, including the Association for Gay Veterinarians (known as PrideVMC today) and the World Federation of Asian Veterinarians, both meeting for the first time in 1978. Minoritized populations within the profession continue to recognize the value and power of building their own communities within the veterinary profession, with the establishment of the Latinx Veterinary Medical Association, National Association for Black Veterinarians, Association of Asian Veterinary Medical Professionals, the Multicultural Veterinary Medical Association, and the like emerging over the last decade or so.

Fortunately, the AVMA and the American Association of Veterinary Medical Colleges (AAVMC) did begin gathering at least race and ethnicity data of veterinary students several decades ago, so we at least have a good grasp of the trends for underrepresented minorities who matriculate into accredited veterinary programs. They also recently started collecting gender identity and sexual orientation data, which we do not cover in this article but which are available in their annual reports.

According to AAVMC in 2023, the racial/ethnic makeup of the students in AVMA-accredited veterinary schools in the United States was approximately 80% white, 8% Latino/Hispanic, 5% Asian, 4% multiracial/multiethnic, 3% African American/Black, and less than 1% Native Hawaiian/Pacific Islander or American Indian/Alaska Native.[21] This is slightly better than what is reported for veterinarians in the field, which, according to the Bureau of Labor Statistics in 2022, was about 91% white, 2% Black, 4% Asian, and 0.5% Hispanic/Latinx. Given that the racial and ethnic makeup of the United States, based on the 2020 census, is approximately 59% white, 19% Hispanic/Latinx, 13% Black/African American, 6% Asian, 2% multiethnic/multiracial, and less than 1% American Indian/Alaska Native or Native Hawaiian/Pacific Islander, the profession is lagging, and while student numbers are improving, it is still paltry compared with the overall makeup of the United States' population.[22] This is particularly true for those who identify as African American/Black and Latinx/Hispanic—who make up 12% and 19% of the current US population, respectively, according to the 2020 census.

This background information provides a segue into understanding the reasons that specialty medicine lacks diversity, as well. Of course, when there are fewer in the pool, it is less likely that they will go on to obtain further training. But there are other issues at play, too. Without role models, it is difficult to even imagine yourself standing there; we know this to be true from research that clearly demonstrates the importance of representation in all walks of life. And, of course, there are the implicit and overt biases that exist when assessing application packets. The research is also clear that ethnic-sounding names, gender, and other biases persist when making selections for jobs, scholarships, awards, and a variety of other sought-after positions/roles. Why should this be any different for board-certified specialists in veterinary medicine?

Before we dive too deeply into the numbers, let us first provide you a brief historical overview of the veterinary specialty colleges in the United States. Preventive Medicine and Pathology were the first formally founded veterinary specialties, both forming in 1950. The formation of these two specialties gave rise to the Advisory Board on Veterinary Specialties (ABVS) after applications from the American College of Veterinary Pathologists and the American Board of Veterinary Public Health applied to be recognized as specialty organizations. In 1951, the AVMA, which has been in existence since 1863, approved both the criteria for recognizing veterinary specialty organizations and the specialties in public health (which later became the American College of Veterinary Preventive Medicine) and pathology.[23]

Currently, the ABVS recognizes 22 veterinary specialty organizations, made up of 46 distinct specialties.[24] About 14% of veterinarians have earned diplomate status, equivalent to about 16,500 veterinarians in the United States. Although many of these Colleges have diversity committees and may be working to collect such data, unlike the veterinary student and US veterinarian populations, no data regarding the diversity—of any kind—of these specialties are currently widely available. Thus, it is almost impossible to even estimate the gender, religious, sexual orientation, or ethnic diversity within each College or within the specialty community as a whole. This is not terribly surprising, however, given that the veterinary colleges themselves did not seek to collect or collate this information until 1980, although the AAVMC has been collecting student data from its member institutions since the early 1970s.

Unfortunately, there is no organization that has stepped up to collect similar data about the specialty organizations. While there are estimates of how many veterinarians are board-certified and each College has a record of the Diplomates they have certified, the numbers generally end there. Thus, there is relatively little information that is readily available regarding specialists that were or are members of groups that have been historically marginalized. This is as true of the very first specialty colleges as it is of the newest, and attempts to find information about historically marginalized individuals in any of the Colleges were thwarted by either lack of data or outright anger.

It does appear likely that Dr Eugene Adams was the first boarded pathologist. While the specific date he earned this designation was not openly available, it is estimated that he earned his board certification status sometime in the early 1960s, which coincides with the completion of his graduate studies at Cornell University, which he began in 1955.[25] For the American College of Veterinary Preventive Medicine, we were unable to determine who was the first non-white boarded diplomate, despite reaching out to numerous individuals within the College to seek this information. Nor were we able to glean any other demographic information about their 900 current and 300 emeritus diplomates.

There are some specialty colleges for which there are lists of Black/African American diplomates, as Dr Patterson turned an idea into something bigger in 2023 and was able to collect the names of these individuals for the American College of Veterinary Internal

Medicine (ACVIM) for internal medicine, cardiology, neurology, and oncology: the American College of Dermatology, and the American College of Ophthalmology.[26] The collection of this information started because of Dr Patterson's desire to recognize a colleague during Black History Month in 2022, Dr Erick Mears, with whom she had shared mentors and career paths. When she reached out to the ACVIM to establish when he had become board certified, she became curious about how many other Black internists there were and discovered that the information was not being collected, so she did it herself and passed it onto the ACVIM membership manager. She later decided to reach out to other specialties to see if they were collecting this information; it turns out, none of them were and most still do not.[26]

However, other specialty colleges have since started seeking diversity information from their members. The American College of Veterinary Emergency and Critical Care Diversity Committee published a paper in 2020 outlining the organization's steps to enhance diversity, equity, and inclusion (DEI) within its ranks.[27] They also started several other initiatives, including a demographics survey along with providing training by offering the Purdue University Diversity and Inclusion Certificate, to members at a discount.[27] And in 2021, the American College of Veterinary Surgeons (ACVS) sent a survey out to members seeking to gather demographic information on their diplomates and to summarize perspectives on the importance of DEI initiatives.[28] After analyzing the data, the authors concluded that "despite strong support for DEI from most respondents, some diplomates stated or insinuated that initiatives to increase diversity threaten the quality of candidates and future surgeons and found this to be of particular concern. Further, there appeared to be concerns related to gender inequalities, sexism, and misogyny within our specialty. Targeted efforts to include DEI as part of the mission of the ACVS, as well as efforts to address workplace culture and climate and pipelines, should be emphasized."[28(p1852)]

It is important to note that the American College of Laboratory Animal Medicine and American College of Veterinary Pathologists have also created DEI committees. Although there are no currently published reports on their activities and/or initiatives that we could find, we understand they have been working to create training and collect demographic information on their members.

As already stated, representation matters. This is as true of the veterinary profession writ large as it is of the specialty colleges; if applicants to internship and residency training programs continue to be selected as they have always been, the perpetuation of underrepresentation will continue. This is borne out by research by Chun and colleagues,[20] who noted that faculty in veterinary medical colleges tend to mirror the overall demographics of the profession. And in the 2022 Veterinary Intern and Residency Matching Program data set, it is notable that applicants tend to also mirror the demographics of the profession, despite slight increases in numbers of students identifying as members of historically marginalized groups. Chun and colleagues[29(p421)] also describe several factors that have thwarted efforts at improving diversity and suggest methods to ameliorate these, including the following:

1. Using consistent criteria to assess each candidate rather than relying on "best fit" with the program.
2. If GPA is used during selection, identifying the courses contributing to the calculation, recognizing the lack of consistency among schools/colleges, and determining whether the applicant's grades improved over time during their DVM training.
3. If considering class rank, recognizing the challenges associated with this metric due to the actual grades of each applicant being slightly variable.

4. Looking for extracurricular activities, especially those outside veterinary medicine (sports, music, performing arts, and so forth); these may be additional indicators of professional success.

Chun and colleagues[29(p422)] end with a charge to the schools and colleges of veterinary medicine: "each institution must develop and nurture safe avenues for discussion of these important topics within all levels of the organization, along with support and provision of continuing education and professional development opportunities that foster inclusive behaviors, a deep understanding of the impact of bias within the organization, and the value of hiring and training individuals with diverse backgrounds and attributes. Each school and college must practice shared governance and a way for all stakeholders to have an opportunity to voice their perspectives during major decisions. DEI must always be a priority. In addition to an improved focus on diversity, equity and inclusiveness in student selection, the same considerations must be intentionally included during intern, resident, staff, and faculty recruitment. While the principles are the same, the benefits can be truly profound and determine an organization's success well into the future. It must be made clear throughout the organization that policies are explicitly in place to support DEI initiatives and strategies."

We, the authors of this article, echo this charge. This is an inflection point for our profession. We are experiencing unprecedented shortages in nearly every facet. We have 15 new colleges on the horizon and already face significant faculty shortages in the current accredited US veterinary colleges. The profession *must* change how it has engaged with people from historically marginalized backgrounds. We owe it to ourselves and the stakeholders that we serve. We can and must do better!

DISCLOSURE

The authors have nothing to disclose.

Coretta Patterson, DVM, DACVIM(SA), PG Cert Vet Med Ed
College of Veterinary Medicine
Midwestern University
Downers Grove, IL, USA

Katherine Fogelberg, DVM, PhD (Science Education)
Thrive Pet Healthcare

E-mail addresses:
cpatte2@midwestern.edu (C. Patterson)
katherine.fogelberg@thrivepet.com (K. Fogelberg)

REFERENCES

1. Oxford Languages. Available at: www.google.com. Accessed August 5, 2024.
2. Cooper LA, Beach MC, Johnson RL, et al. Delving below the surface: understanding how race and ethnicity influence relationships in health care. J Gen Intern Med 2005;21(Suppl 1):S21–7. https://doi.org/10.1111/j.1525-1497.2006. 00305.x.
3. Moore C, Coates E, Watson A, et al. "It's important to work with people that look like me": Black patients' preferences for patient-provider race-concordance. J Racial Ethn Health Disparities 2022;10:2552–64. https://doi.org/10.1007/s40615-022-01435-y.

4. Komarmomy M, Grumbacj K, Drake M, et al. The role of Black and Hispanic physicians in providing health care for underserved populations. New Engl J Med 1996;334(20):1305–10.

5. Cohen JJ, Gabriel BA, Terrell C. The case for diversity in the health care workforce. Health Affairs 2010;21(5):90–102. https://doi.org/10.1377/hlthaff.21.21.5.90.

6. Meghani AH, Brooks JM, Gipson-Jones T, et al. Patient-provider race-concordance: does it matter in improving minority patients' health outcomes? Ethn Health 2009;14(1):107–30.

7. Simonds VW, Christopher S, Sequist TD, et al. Exploring patient-provider interactions in a Native American community. J Health Care Poor Underserved 2011; 22(3):836–52.

8. Jang Y, Yoon H, Kim MT, et al. Preference for patient–provider ethnic concordance in Asian Americans. Ethnicity Health 2021;26(3):448–59.

9. State University College of Veterinary Medicine. (n.d.). History. Available at: www. vetmed.iastate.edu/about/history. (Accessed 2 August 2024).

10. Gill G, Singh B. Where do deans of veterinary medicine in the United States and Canada come from? Can Vet J 2020;61(11):1187–96. Available at: https://www. ncbi.nlm.nih.gov/pmc/articles/PMC7560764/. Accessed August 9, 2024.

11. Vezeau N, Kemelmakher H, Seixas JS, et al. Characterizing global gender representation in veterinary executive leadership. J Vet Med Educ 2024. https://doi. org/10.3138/jvme-2023-0092 (advance access article).

12. Tynan A. Veterinarians with disabilities: an international issue. J Vet Med Educ 2004;31(1):22–7.

13. Cima G. Legends: America's first DVM, Daniel E. Salmon helped reduce disease in animals and humans. 2013. Available at: https://www.avma.org/javma-news/ 2013-03-01/legends-americas-first-dvm. Accessed August 4, 2024.

14. American Veterinary Medical Association. Diversity timeline: evolution of a profession. 2020. Available at: https://www.avma.org/javma-news/2010-02-15/diversity-timeline. Accessed August 4, 2024.

15. Cornell University College of Veterinary Medicine. Celebrating women's history month. 2024. Available at: https://www.vet.cornell.edu/celebrating-womens-history-month. Accessed August 2, 2024.

16. University of Missouri Zalk Veterinary Medical Library. Black veterinary history: Augustus Nathaniel Lushington. 2018. Available at: https://libraryguides.missouri. edu/AfricanAmericanVeterinaryHistory/Lushington. Accessed August 2, 2024.

17. University of Missouri Zalk Veterinary Medical Library. Black veterinary history: Dr Alfreda Johnson Webb. 2018. Available at: https://libraryguides.missouri.edu/ AfricanAmericanVeterinaryHistory/JohnsonWebb. Accessed August 2, 2024.

18. Association for Women in Science. Dr Jane Hinton, PhD. 2024. Available at: https://awis.org/historical-women/dr-jane-hinton/. Accessed August 4, 2024.

19. Kahler SC. Women's organization nurtured, influenced. American Veterinary Medical Association. 2013. Available at: https://www.avma.org/javma-news/2013-10-01/womens-organization-nurtured-influenced#:~:text=Chartered%20as%20the %20Women's%20Veterinary,were%20doing%2C%E2%80%9D%20said%20Dr. Accessed August 9, 2024.

20. PrideVMC. PrideVMC has a long and storied 30+ years of history. It grew out of the gay liberation events following Stonewall in 1977. Available at: https:// pridevmc.org/history/. Accessed August 9, 2024.

21. American Association of Veterinary Medical Colleges. Annual data report. 2023. Available at: https://www.aavmc.org/wp-content/uploads/2023/09/2023-AAVMC-Annual-Data-Report-September23.pdf. Accessed August 4, 2024.

22. Childers L. It takes a village: supporting DEIB efforts in the veterinary field. American Animal Hospital Association; 2023. Available at: https://www.vetmed.ucdavis.edu/news/it-takes-village#:~:text=According%20to%202022%20data%20from,0.5%25%20are%20Hispanic%2FLatinx. Accessed August 4, 2024.

23. Larkin M. A visual history of the AVMA's first 150 years. 2013. Available at: https://www.avma.org/javma-news/2013-07-15/one-history-books. Accessed August 5, 2024.

24. American Board of Veterinary Specialties. Veterinary specialties. 2024. Available at: https://www.avma.org/education/veterinary-specialties. Accessed August 5, 2024.

25. Kansas State University College of Veterinary Medicine. History: Prominent African Americans in veterinary medicine. Available at: https://www.vet.k-state.edu/about/diversity/history-aa.html. Accessed August 5, 2024.

26. Larkin M. List of Black diplomates sparks discussion, action. Dr. Coretta Patterson took on a passion project to highlight and encourage diversity in veterinary specialty colleges. 2023. Available at: https://avmajournals.avma.org/display/post/news/list-of-black-diplomates-sparks-discussion–action.xml. Accessed August 4, 2024.

27. Odunayo A, Alwood A, Asokan V, et al. Our quest for creating a space that is welcoming to all: A commentary from the American College of Veterinary Emergency and Critical Care diversity, equity, and inclusion committee. J Vet Emerg Crit Care 2022;32:165–7. https://doi.org/10.1111/vec.13190.

28. Gonzalez LM, Stampley AR, Marcellin-Little DJ, et al. Respondents to an American College of Veterinary Surgeons diplomate survey support the promotion of diversity, equity, and inclusion initiatives. J Am Vet Med Assoc 2023;261(12):1847–52. https://doi.org/10.2460/javma.23.06.0310.

29. Chun R, Davis E, Frank N, et al. Can veterinary medicine improve diversity in post-graduate training programs? Current state of academic veterinary medicine and recommendations on best practices. J Am Vet Med Assoc 2023;261(3):417–23. https://doi.org/10.2460/javma.22.09.0430.

Bridging Gaps in Veterinary Care: Equity, Access, and Innovation

Michael Blackwell, DVM, MPH

KEYWORDS

- Health equity • Access to veterinary care • DEI • Incremental care
- Spectrum of care • One health

KEY POINTS

- Health inequity threatens the well-being of pets, families, and veterinary care teams.
- All who wish to enjoy companionship with a pet deserve to have it and need access to veterinary care.
- To ensure access to veterinary care, innovations in veterinary service delivery are paramount.

COMPASSIONATE CARE AT THE CROSSROADS OF SOCIOECONOMIC REALITIES

Pause for a moment to visualize a scenario tinged with somber reflection rather than celebration. Consider the life of an elderly woman, a retired public servant whose career as a librarian enriched countless individuals in her community. Now, in the tranquil latter years of her life, she faces a formidable challenge. Her cherished cat, a steadfast companion throughout her serene retirement, has fallen severely ill. The exorbitant cost of necessary medical treatment cast a long, dark shadow over their future together, ultimately leading to the heart-wrenching decision to euthanize, as the financial burden posed an insurmountable barrier to recovery.

This painful decision to part with her beloved pet is not a choice made willingly but a forced concession to overwhelming financial constraints. It starkly highlights the deficiencies in a societal system that often fails to support those who have dedicated their lives to public service, now struggling to make ends meet in their golden years. The isolation experienced by seniors living alone poses a significant threat to their mental and emotional well-being, underscoring the urgent need for supportive community networks and resources.[1]

Declaration of AI and AI Assisted Technologies in the Writing Process: During the preparation of this work the author used ChatGPT Creative Writer to assist with clarity and the overall flow. After using this tool, the author reviewed and edited the content as needed and takes full responsibility for the content of the publication.

Program for Pet Health Equity, The University of Tennessee, 600 Henley Street, Suite 221, Knoxville, TN 37996, USA

E-mail address: mblackw1@utk.edu

As we strive for excellence in veterinary medicine, this narrative should serve as a poignant reminder of the profound impact our profession has on the lives of the individuals and families we serve. It compels us to confront a disturbing question: How does our current societal framework fail to maintain the integrity of family units when access to essential veterinary care is beyond reach?

Across the nation, pets are more than just animals; they are integral members of families.

Nearly all US pet owners (97%) say their pets are part of their family, and about half of them (51%) not only consider their pets to be a part of their family but say they are *as much a part of their family as a human member.*[2] However, the critical bonds that integrate pets into these familial networks are frequently jeopardized, not by choice, but by daunting socioeconomic barriers—predominantly financial constraints. This reality can dismantle the cherished sense of companionship and belonging, replacing it with a void filled with loss and solitude. We must thoughtfully consider our role within the veterinary industry: How can we collaboratively enhance our services to bridge gaps rather than widen them—fostering healing and unity among families rather than exacerbating divisions due to unequal access?

The narrative of our retired librarian is not unique but a reflection of a widespread issue—a narrative shared by many families grappling with similar challenges. This scenario sheds light on a broader societal issue of disparities in health care access that significantly affects numerous families with pets. Recognizing that the wellness of pets is deeply intertwined with the emotional and physical health of their families, it is imperative that the provision of veterinary care be regarded not as a luxury but as an essential service within a compassionate society. The bond we share with our pets surpasses mere companionship; it is a fundamental aspect of family life that demands recognition and protection. This relationship transcends societal divides, offering joy, therapeutic support, and steadfast companionship amidst life's challenges.

As veterinary professionals, affirming this bond commits us to its defense and promotion.

This awareness should inspire us to action. Our responsibilities begin with acknowledging this fundamental relationship and extend into proactive efforts to transform our industry. Now is the time to turn our commitments into a dynamic force for change, ensuring no pet suffers due to financial constraints—a mission inherently linked to compassion, justice, and the ethical foundation of veterinary practice.

As we commit to the principles of diversity, equity, and inclusion (DEI) within veterinary medicine, we must clearly define our ultimate objective: health equity. Health equity is the condition in which every individual, irrespective of their race, gender, ethnicity, or background, has the opportunity to reach their full health potential without facing disadvantages. This means ensuring that all people have fair and impartial access to health care services, including veterinary care, necessary to achieve optimal health outcomes. Achieving equity requires a genuine commitment to inclusion, acknowledging that a "one-size-fits-all" approach is ineffective in our diverse society. Inclusion in veterinary care means actively developing and implementing service delivery systems that are specifically tailored to meet the cultural, economic, and social needs of the various families we serve. Inclusion necessitates the creation of a diverse range of services tailored to accommodate varying financial capabilities, cultural practices, and the unique living conditions of families with pets, ensuring equitable access to quality care, free from bias or barriers.

To operationalize DEI principles effectively, we must engage in a continuous dialogue with the communities we serve, asking pertinent questions and listening intently to their needs and experiences. This dialogue helps us to identify and understand the barriers that prevent access to care and compels us to take proactive steps to dismantle these obstacles. Our strategies must be adaptable, evolving as we gain insights and feedback from our efforts. This means not only adjusting our existing services but also innovating new ones that bridge gaps in care. Every action taken should move us closer to a veterinary health care system where equity is the norm, and every pet and their family receives the care they need to thrive.

Let us strive toward a future where the strength of enduring bonds is not threatened by socioeconomic strife, and each call for aid is met with understanding and effective support. We envision a world where veterinary care surpasses the mere provision of services for animals and symbolizes a societal ethos that respects and cherishes all life equally, ensuring no distinction between the affluent and the underserved. This embodies a system finely attuned to the varied economic realities of individuals, poised to offer equitable and respectful care to every member of the community, both human and animal.

UNDERSTANDING ACCESS TO VETERINARY HEALTH CARE AS A FUNDAMENTAL RIGHT

Access to health care, critical for both humans and animals, entails more than the availability of services; it encompasses the capacity of individuals or communities to utilize essential medical services that are timely, affordable, and appropriate. Recognized universally as a fundamental component of public health and a basic human right, comprehensive access is essential for fostering health and well-being across all populations. This concept holds particular significance in veterinary medicine, highlighting the various social and environmental factors that impact how individuals care for their pets in their daily environments.

To gain a full understanding of access within veterinary care, it is helpful to examine the framework presented by Penchansky and Thomas,[3] known as the "5 A's" of access to care:

1. Affordability: Veterinary services are priced within the financial reach of all families.
2. Availability: Sufficient veterinary resources and care points are readily available to meet the needs of all families.
3. Accessibility: Families can easily travel to and access veterinary facilities.
4. Accommodation: Veterinary services are structured and scheduled to align with the diverse constraints and preferences of families.
5. Acceptability: Families feel comfortable with the veterinary provider's fundamental cultural norms, ensuring mutual respect and understanding.

To address the unique challenges within veterinary medicine, the traditional framework of the "5 A's of access to care" is expanded with 2 additional dimensions:

6. Awareness: Enhancing health education and outreach efforts to ensure that families understand the importance of veterinary care.
7. Health information systems: Implementing comprehensive IT systems that facilitate holistic care coordination across family health care needs.

As members of the veterinary profession, we are bound by a profound oath[4]—a pledge to use our scientific knowledge and skills to benefit society, extending far beyond the confines of our clinics. This covenant emphasizes our commitment not only to the health and welfare of our patients but equally to the humans whose lives are intimately connected with theirs. Our unified pledge, to serve, protect, and heal all without prejudice, reaches into the very heart of society, affirming that our responsibilities extend beyond individual care to encompass broader social implications. This pledge is unwavering in its inclusivity, making no exceptions based on financial capacity or economic standing. It steadfastly commits to serving every member of our diverse community, not just the privileged.

A significant challenge within veterinary care is the persistent belief that having a pet is a privilege reserved for those who can afford the associated costs. While concerns for animal welfare underpin this viewpoint, it overlooks the substantial emotional and health benefits pets provide.[5] It becomes imperative for the veterinary profession to actively address these disparities. Especially crucial is the recognition that individuals with limited financial resources may benefit most profoundly from the companionship and well-being pets provide. Veterinary professionals must therefore transcend traditional judgments and innovate, developing accessible health care solutions that cater to all pets and their families. By doing so, veterinarians affirm that the emotional and physical benefits pets offer should be universally accessible, particularly to those in society who need them the most.

The Access to Veterinary Care Coalition (AVCC), formed in early 2016, drew attention to the problem of lack of access to veterinary care. The AVCC worked in association with the University of Tennessee College of Social Work and College of Veterinary Medicine, to conduct a national study (made possible by the generosity of Maddie's Fund) of pet owners, including populations with inadequate access to veterinary care, and veterinary service providers. The purpose of the study was to identify barriers that households face, as well as best practices among those delivering veterinary care to underserved pet owners. The results were reported in the seminal document, *Access to Veterinary Care: Barriers, Current Practices, and Public Policy*.[6] The report has been widely disseminated to help guide veterinarians, animal welfare organizations, legislators, community leaders, and others, as they seek to improve access to veterinary care for pets currently without it.

A pivotal study by the AVCC uncovered a troubling crisis: a significant proportion of families, 28% according to the survey, encountered obstacles to accessing veterinary care over the past 2 years (**Fig. 1**). Although financial limitations were frequently cited

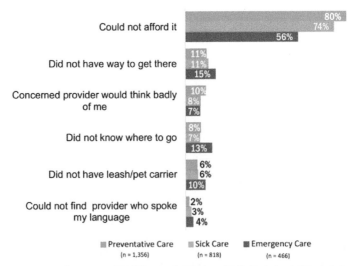

Fig. 1. Barriers to veterinary care (AVCC Report). (Blackwell MJ, Krebsbach SB, et al. Access to Veterinary Care: Barriers, Current Practices, and Public Policy. TRACE: Tennessee Research and Creative Exchange. https://trace.tennessee.edu/utk_smalpubs/17. Published December 17, 2018.)

as the primary hurdle to receiving necessary care, the issue extends beyond mere economic factors and reflects broader societal challenges. Currently, a subsequent survey is underway, expected to reveal that the effects of the COVID-19 pandemic coupled with constraints in the veterinary workforce have likely intensified these barriers.

Veterinarians involved in the AVCC study demonstrated a commitment to serving underserved pets, with 470 participants depicted in **Fig. 2**. Nearly all of these practitioners, accounting for 98.4% of those surveyed, had adopted at least one financial strategy over the previous year to better meet these needs. The predominant approach involved discussing a range of treatment possibilities with clients, while also frequently providing information on available payment options.

In 2018, 29% of US households identified as Asset Limited, Income Constrained, Employed (ALICE), having financial vulnerabilities despite steady employment.[7] ALICE households make up the essential workforce, including retail, food service, construction, agriculture, among other service jobs. Combined with households below the Federal Poverty Level (FPL), a total of 42% struggle to make ends meet. Millennials without a college education earn less than their counterparts in prior generations.[8] These statistics paint a clear picture: access to veterinary care is not just a current issue but is likely to intensify.

The financial burden experienced by families when pet care exceeds affordability can lead to profound moral distress[9] among veterinary professionals who regularly face such economic barriers. They often find themselves torn between their desire to provide care and the economic realities that restrict their capabilities, affecting both the quality of care delivered and the family's emotional well-being. It is imperative that educational programs for veterinary professionals evolve to equip them with the skills necessary to navigate these complex ethical landscapes, ensuring they can blend medical expertise with an understanding of socioeconomic challenges. Also, the veterinary service delivery systems should innately One Health, including allied disciplines, for example, Veterinary Social Work, to served families more holistically.

Envision a society where access to veterinary services is recognized not as a privilege, but as a fundamental right that transcends socioeconomic barriers. As veterinary professionals reflect on their responsibilities, let them be continually reminded of the need to be attentive to the requirements of every family. In reaffirming the foundational values of our oath, the veterinary community must demonstrate unwavering

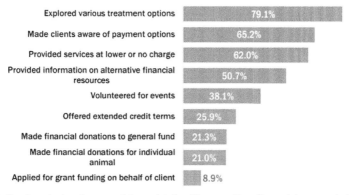

Fig. 2. Methods veterinarians used to assist families needing financial support. (Blackwell MJ, Krebsbach SB, et al. Access to Veterinary Care: Barriers, Current Practices, and Public Policy. TRACE: Tennessee Research and Creative Exchange. https://trace.tennessee.edu/utk_smalpubs/17. Published December 17, 2018.)

determination and clear purpose. The goal is to expand the reach of veterinary care, honoring the profession's commitment to society in its entirety, ensuring that no animal suffers due to financial constraints, and upholding the bond that pets and their families rely on. As veterinary professionals, we are called not just to recognize these challenges but to actively forge paths toward a more equitable future.

INNOVATIVE STRATEGIES FOR ENHANCING VETERINARY CARE: INTEGRATING THE SPECTRUM OF CARE AND INCREMENTAL CARE

In the realm of veterinary medicine, ensuring comprehensive and adaptable patient management, especially under financial constraints, requires an integrated approach that encompasses both the spectrum of care (SoC) and incremental care (IC) (**Fig. 3**). These two frameworks are essential in tailoring treatment plans to the varied needs and financial capacities of pet families. These frameworks are not just methodologies, they are philosophies that fundamentally redefine the engagement and delivery of veterinary services. Let us explore what each of these approaches entails and why their combined application is crucial for delivering effective veterinary care even when resources are limited.

SoC offers a comprehensive model that encompasses all facets of veterinary services—from preventive measures and routine wellness care to advanced surgical procedures and cutting-edge treatments. This broad framework allows veterinary professionals to tailor medical interventions to the specific needs and circumstances of each patient, ensuring that care is available, appropriate, and adaptable.

For example, consider the management of a leg fracture in a dog, which can vary widely depending on the severity and location of the fracture, as well as the dog's age and overall health. SoC allows veterinarians to offer a range of treatment options tailored to these factors. Initial treatments might include stabilization with a splint or cast, pain management with medications, and restricted activity to allow for natural healing. For more complex fractures, surgical options could involve the use of pins, plates, or screws to properly align and secure the bone fragments, followed by physical therapy to aid in recovery.

In addition to these medical treatments, the SoC approach considers the family's financial situation and emotional readiness to engage in postoperative care, which

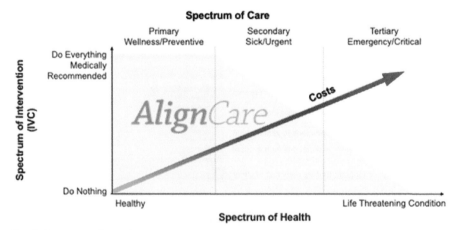

Fig. 3. Incremental veterinary care versus spectrum of care.

might include regular follow ups and adjustments in treatment as the healing process progresses. By integrating a flexible array of therapeutic strategies, veterinary professionals can ensure that each pet receives the most appropriate care while accommodating the diverse circumstances of their families.

IC advocates a meticulous, step-by-step approach to treatment, particularly important in managing long-term conditions or in emergency situations where immediate, extensive interventions may be financially or practically untenable. IC promotes a phased treatment protocol, which can be adjusted based on the patient's response and the client's capacity to manage costs. This strategy encourages a dynamic and reciprocal interaction between the veterinarian and pet family, ensuring decisions are made with a thorough understanding of both medical outcomes and personal constraints (contextualized care).

Imagine a scenario where a cat presents with gastrointestinal symptoms, weight loss, and intermittent vomiting. The symptoms and physical examination suggest possible inflammatory bowel disease (IBD) or an underlying infection, both of which require distinct approaches for diagnosis and treatment. Given limited resources, the veterinarian must use IC to judiciously decide which diagnostics and treatments to prioritize. Initially, the veterinarian opts for basic blood work and fecal tests rather than more expensive imaging studies like an ultrasound. This approach prioritizes tests that can quickly rule out infections or other common issues without incurring higher costs.

Based on the initial test results, the veterinarian begins with conservative management, such as dietary changes and basic medications to stabilize the cat's condition. These interventions are chosen as they are cost-effective and can address a broad spectrum of potential issues.

As the treatment progresses, the cat's response to the dietary and medical management is monitored closely. If there is no improvement, the need for further diagnostics like an ultrasound might be reconsidered. However, more expensive tests or invasive procedures like biopsies, which could definitively diagnose IBD, are delayed until they are absolutely necessary or until more funds become available.

Throughout this process, the veterinarian continuously assesses which treatments are essential for maintaining the cat's quality of life and which can be postponed without jeopardizing their health. This dynamic management ensures that resources are used effectively, with a focus on therapies and diagnostics that offer the greatest benefit relative to their cost at each stage of the cat's treatment.

This strategic approach highlights how veterinary professionals must balance immediate care needs with financial constraints, adapting the treatment plan based on the evolving health status of the pet and the economic reality of the pet's family.

The role of educators and mentors in veterinary medicine extends beyond imparting knowledge of patient care techniques. It is crucial to instill an understanding of how to seamlessly integrate SoC and IC into daily practice. This includes training in effective client communication, ethical decision-making, and handling complex cases that require nuanced, multifaceted strategies.

If SoC is envisioned as a comprehensive map, outlining all possible routes and destinations, then IC acts as a precise navigating tool, guiding each decision along the path. Together, these methodologies not only elevate the standards of veterinary practice but also ensure that it is conducted with integrity, considering the diverse needs and constraints of the communities served.

Thus, the veterinary community is encouraged to fully embrace these nuanced methodologies. Integrating the adaptable scope of the SoC with the thoughtful, patient-centric approach of IC will elevate the standards of veterinary practice, ensuring that treatments are both effective and empathetically aligned with the financial and emotional capacities of pet owners. This comprehensive approach fosters a more inclusive and accessible health care environment, enhancing patient outcomes and satisfaction across diverse pet populations.

REINFORCING OUR MORAL OBLIGATIONS IN VETERINARY CARE

In the words of Dr. Martin Luther King Jr., "The time is always right to do what is right." This profound statement, spoken at Oberlin College in 1964,[10] underscores the enduring relevance of moral courage and integrity, particularly in the face of challenging circumstances. In the context of veterinary medicine, it calls upon us to uphold the highest ethical standards, especially when addressing the complexities associated with providing equitable care.

Embodying this principle means ensuring that all members of our community, regardless of their financial situation or any other barrier, have access to necessary veterinary services. Doing what is right involves more than just treating animals, it requires us to dismantle the systemic barriers that prevent families from receiving adequate care. This commitment to justice and equity in veterinary care not only honors Dr. King's legacy but also deepens our professional resolve to serve every pet and their family with compassion and respect.

Facing such challenges head-on, veterinary care teams must innovate and advocate for policies and practices that extend care to underserved populations. It is in these actions—striving to provide the best possible care to all, advocating for policy changes, and educating communities about animal health—that we truly embody the call to do what is right, turning Dr. King's words into actionable change within our field.

Reflecting on Dr. King's profound insights reminds us that our profession embodies a deeper societal role, not merely confined to medical treatment but entwined with higher moral and ethical responsibilities. Veterinary medicine, with its unique blend of science and compassion, calls us to act with courage in the face of adversity, to lead with integrity amid uncertainty, and to advocate passionately for those without a voice.

Today, our profession stands at a significant crossroads, facing the choice between the comfort of familiar paths and the challenge of less trodden routes. These less familiar paths, though fraught with challenges, are illuminated by the potential for significant positive impact and are paved with the principles of justice and compassion. Choosing this route requires not just skill and knowledge, but a deep-seated bravery to push beyond conventional boundaries and effect real change.

In this transformative era, educators, practitioners, and pioneers in veterinary medicine are called upon to foster a new ethical framework—one that infuses a moral compass into every aspect of veterinary practice. This new ethos should guide our students and colleagues to not only excel in their clinical skills but also to practice with a profound sense of justice and empathy.

The disparities present in pet health care often reflect broader societal inequalities that affect marginalized and underserved populations. Tackling these disparities requires a committed approach to inclusivity, ensuring that every veterinary student and professional is equipped to provide compassionate and competent care across economic, racial, and cultural divides. By doing so, we prepare them to serve a broader demographic, addressing the needs of all community members and their pets with the same high standard of care.

Our dedication to the future of veterinary medicine must encompass more than the transmission of knowledge and technical skills. It is imperative that we cultivate within ourselves the ability to confront and navigate complex ethical dilemmas that we will inevitably face in practice. We must instill the courage to make difficult decisions that reflect both medical ethics and social justice, ensuring we are well prepared to serve our communities with both expertise and empathy.

As we reflect on our role and the legacy we wish to build, we extend a call to action to each member of the veterinary community to ponder deeply what we are contributing to the fabric of society. Let us unite in a solemn pledge to ensure that our efforts in veterinary education and practice not only serve as beacons of hope but also as models of comprehensive health and justice. Together, let us forge ahead with a shared commitment to a future where veterinary medicine not only meets the immediate needs of animals but also addresses the broader societal challenges, reflecting a deep collective conscience and an unwavering commitment to all forms of life.

DISCLOSURE

There is nothing to disclose.

FUNDING

Maddie's Fund is acknowleged.

REFERENCES

1. Roy K, Smilowitz S, Bhatt S, et al. Impact of social isolation and loneliness in older adults: current understanding and future directions. Curr Geri Rep 2023;12:138–48.
2. Brown A. About half of U.S. pet owners say their pets are as much a part of their family as a human member. Pew Research Center. 2023. Available at: https://www.pewresearch.org/short-reads/2023/07/07/about-half-us-of-pet-owners-say-their-pets-are-as-much-a-part-of-their-family-as-a-human-member/.
3. Penchansky R, Thomas JW. The concept of access: definition and relationship to consumer satisfaction. Med Care 1981;19(2):127–40.
4. American Veterinary Medicine Association, Veterinarian's Oath. Available at: https://www.avma.org/resources-tools/avma-policies/veterinarians-oath.
5. Hussein SM, Soliman WS, Khalifa AA. Benefits of pets' ownership, a review based on health perspectives. J Intern Med 2021;2(1):1–9.
6. Blackwell MJ, Krebsbach SB, et al. Access to veterinary care: barriers, current practices, and public policy. TRACE: tennessee research and creative exchange. Available at: https://trace.tennessee.edu/utk_smalpubs/17. Accessed December 17, 2018.
7. United For ALICE. Available at: https://unitedforalice.org/meet-alice?gad_source=1.
8. Bialik K, Fry R. Millenial Life: How young adulthood today compares with prior generations. Pew Research Center. 2019. Available at: https://www.pewresearch.org/social-trends/2019/02/14/millennial-life-how-young-adulthood-today-compares-with-prior-generations-2/.
9. Jameton A. What moral distress in nursing history could suggest about the future of health care. AMA J Ethics 2017;19(6):617–28.
10. Dr. Martin Luther King, Jr., The future of Integration. Oberlin College Achieves. Available at: https://www2.oberlin.edu/external/EOG/BlackHistoryMonth/MLK/MLKmainpage.html.

Inclusive Mentorship for the Next Generation of Veterinary Professionals

Marie Sato Quicksall, DVM, CVA*

KEYWORDS

- Inclusion • Mentorship • Veterinary medicine
- BIPOC (black, indigenous, people of color)
- LGBTQIA+ (lesbian, gay, bisexual, queer, intersex, asexual, plus) • Gender

KEY POINTS

- Inclusive mentorship has the potential to increase representation and retention of BIPOC individuals in the field.
- Inclusive mentorship can benefit mentees, mentors, the profession, and society at large.
- Successful and inclusive mentoring relationships include good communication, trust, and psychological safety.
- Creating an inclusive environment before beginning mentorship relationships increases the chances of success.
- Incorporate inclusion into program design, mentor training, and ongoing maintenance of mentoring relationships.

INTRODUCTION

Mentorship plays a large role in the veterinary profession. When done in a constructive way, mentorship has the potential to address multiple shortfalls and concerns in the veterinary field. Veterinary medicine is one of the least diverse fields in the country in terms of race and ethnicity, with 90% of veterinarians, 89.8% of veterinary technicians, and 85.7% of veterinary assistants identifying as white.[1] Inclusive mentorship has the potential to shift this lack of diversity and benefit both the profession and society at large.

DEFINITIONS: WHAT IS INCLUSIVE MENTORSHIP?

Mentorship has multiple definitions and multiple types. Henry-Noel and colleagues,[2] in their article "Mentorship in Medicine and Other Health Professions," define mentorship

Multicultural Veterinary Medical Association, PO Box 1742, Silverdale, WA, USA
* Corresponding author.
E-mail address: quicksalldvm@gmail.com

Vet Clin Small Anim 54 (2024) 869–880
https://doi.org/10.1016/j.cvsm.2024.07.014
0195-5616/24/© 2024 Elsevier Inc. All rights reserved, including those for text and data mining, AI training, and similar technologies.
vetsmall.theclinics.com

as "a two-way relationship and type of human development in which one individual invests personal knowledge, energy, and time in order to help another individual grow and develop and improve to become the best and most successful they can be."

Social inclusion is defined "first as the process of improving the terms for individuals and groups to participate in society, and second, as the process of improving the ability, opportunity, and dignity of people, disadvantaged on the basis of their identity, to take part in society."[3]

A mentorship framework that promotes inclusion is critical mentorship. Critical mentorship considers the context of the social identities of both mentors and mentees related to race, ethnicity, gender, sexual orientation, and class. These identities do not have to be shared by the mentors or mentees, but they are a focus of the design and functioning of the mentoring relationship.[4]

WHY IS INCLUSIVE MENTORSHIP IMPORTANT?

Inclusive mentorship has the ability to positively impact not only the individuals in the mentoring relationship but also the veterinary profession and society more broadly.

For the Mentee and Mentor

Effective mentorship can have multiple positive impacts for the mentor and the workplace, particularly when it comes to employee retention and productivity. These effects often stem from the various positive impacts mentees receive from mentoring relationships. Inclusive mentorship can enhance these benefits for marginalized and underrepresented groups. BIPOC (black, indigenous, and people of color) and women are more likely to feel excluded in the workplace, which is linked to lower reported well-being and job dissatisfaction.[5]

Mental health and well-being are common topics of concern in the veterinary field. Studies have linked the meaningful work of veterinary medicine as a positive aspect of the field when it comes to well-being. The 3 components of meaningful work noted in our field include self-actualizing work, helping animals and people, and a sense of belonging.[6] Belonging is defined as a person feeling they are an integral part of a system or environment through their personal involvement in the said system or environment.[7] Inclusive mentorship has been shown to increase reported feelings of belonging.[8–10]

A sense of belonging can also mitigate the effects of stereotype threat.[11–13] Stereotype threat is a psychological threat defined as "being at risk of confirming, as self-characteristic, a negative stereotype about one's group."[14] Individuals with marginalized identities experience stereotype threat when completing a task that is associated with a negative stereotype about their group. These individuals feel that their performance, when completing the said task, will reflect not only upon themselves but also the entire group to which they belong. Stereotype threat can lead to a higher cognitive burden, decreased performance, and increased disengagement.[14–16]

Burnout is also a common concern in veterinary medicine.[17] Mentorship has been shown to decrease burnout for mentees.[18,19] Inclusive mentorship has the potential to decrease burnout specifically for individuals from underrepresented groups.[20,21] A reduction in burnout can lead to higher employee retention.[22,23] For students from underrepresented groups, successful mentorship improves recruitment and retention, whereas poor mentorship contributes to attrition.[24]

Stress can also be increased when individuals experience discrimination based on their social identities, particularly for those early in their veterinary career.[25] Discrimination has been noted in the veterinary field. A 2019 study from the British Veterinary

Association showed 24% of respondents had witnessed or personally experienced discrimination in the prior 12 months.[26]

Mentees also benefit by exposure to different perspectives, philosophies, and mindsets when they are paired with mentors who have different backgrounds from their own.[2,27] Research indicates sharing social identities is not a requirement for effective and inclusive mentorship. Sharing similar attitudes has been shown to be a better predictor of a successful mentoring relationship than shared demographics.[28]

For the Veterinary Profession

As previously noted, veterinary medicine has a lack of representation when it comes to BIPOC. The lack of representation in the field means we are not getting the benefit of various perspectives. When a group includes multiple different perspectives and thinking styles, we can see increased innovation, improved problem solving, and more accurate predictions. This improvement in outcomes is known as the diversity bonus.[29]

We also see that mentorship that improves diversity and representation can have a longer term impact by creating a self-perpetuating cycle of mentorship. Individuals who have been mentored themselves are more likely to go on to become mentors to others.[30]

The experiences that individuals have, particularly during schooling and early in their careers, have an impact on how they view their workplaces, as well as the profession as a whole. Inclusive mentoring relationships and environments can create positive associations and may lead to better retention in the field. Conversely, negative experiences can lead to negative associations, as can be seen with microaggressions. Microaggressions are defined by psychologist Derald Wing Sue[31] as "brief and commonplace daily verbal, behavioral, or environmental indignities, whether intentional or unintentional, that communicate hostile, derogatory, or negative racial slights and insults toward people of color". Originally coined in reference to race and ethnicity, the term microaggression has since expanded to incorporate similar interactions for other marginalized groups. Medical students who experienced frequent microaggressions were more likely to believe microaggressions were a normal part of medical school culture and more likely to consider transfer or withdrawal from their medical school.[32]

For Society

The demographics of the United States are changing. As of 2020, the majority of those younger than 17 years in the United States come from a minority background. As this trend continues, it is projected that the majority of all Americans will come from a minority background by the mid-2040s, known as the "minority majority shift."[33] This shift to less than 50% of the population identifying as white is already seen in the 2020 census in 6 major metropolitan areas, Dallas-Fort Worth, Orlando, Atlanta, Sacramento, New Orleans, and Austin.[34] As we become a more diverse country, it is critical to ensure veterinary medicine is accessible and inclusive to our growing population of BIPOC clients.

Contrary to the common stereotype, BIPOC households own pets at similar rates as white households. In the 2018 *AVMA Pet Ownership and Demographics Sourcebook*, across racial and ethnic groups, a similar percentage of respondents reported their cats and dogs as being family members or companions/pets, indicating the human-animal bond is similarly strong across all racial and ethnic groups.[35]

A 2021 study showed that how pet owners described their relationships with their pets did differ by race and ethnicity. However, race and ethnicity did not affect willingness to seek veterinary care. In addition, black and Native American respondents were more likely to cite lack of trust as a barrier to accessing care for their pet.[36] Another study showed that spaying and neutering of pets was similar across racial and ethnic groups when structural and socioeconomic barriers were removed.[37] Practitioners working in historically underserved communities who reported higher levels of confidence in providing culturally competent care saw an increase in client-provider interactions and utilization of spay-neuter services.[38]

Inclusive mentorship can give both mentees and mentors more exposure to diverse perspectives and experiences. There can be exposure to different lived experiences and cultures when mentors and mentees have different backgrounds, which has the potential to translate to client interactions. Increasing representation of those with marginalized identities in the field can increase the diversity of perspectives. This increased diversity has the potential to increase the exposure of all veterinary professionals to a variety of cultures, perspectives, and experiences, which will increase in our client population as it diversifies.

CHARACTERISTICS OF SUCCESSFUL AND INCLUSIVE MENTORING RELATIONSHIPS

There is a large body of research, particularly in science and medicine, around what makes successful mentoring relationships. Several key themes are found repeatedly in the literature and are directly impacted by inclusivity, or the lack thereof: good communication and trust.[24,39]

Good communication requires being able to communicate openly, honestly, and authentically and having mutual respect.[24,39–41] Psychological safety is important in fostering all of the aforementioned aspects of communication. When individuals feel psychologically safe, they believe they are safe to take interpersonal risk or otherwise be vulnerable in an interpersonal relationship.[42] When medical students felt they had psychological safety in a peer mentoring program, they were able to focus better on their present task and had better relationship building with their mentors.[43] For racialized and otherwise marginalized individuals, psychological safety is important to bring one's open, honest, and authentic self into a mentoring relationship.

When there is a lack of inclusivity and psychological safety, one consequence is identity cover. Individuals with marginalized identities, including BIPOC, women, and LGBTQIA+ (lesbian, gay, bisexual, queer, intersex, asexual, plus) people, often feel pressure to downplay or "cover" their stigmatized identity in an attempt to blend in with the mainstream.[44] Examples include openly gay individuals refraining from bringing their same sex partners to work events and BIPOC individuals avoiding workplace resource groups for fear of being defined solely by their race. Most individuals who reported covering in the workplace felt an expectation to cover from leadership. This expectation affected their sense of available opportunities, as well as their sense of commitment to the organization. These individuals also felt covering was detrimental to their sense of self.[45] Identity cover can be a barrier to open and authentic communication.

Self-reflection in a mentoring relationship is also a key component to both good communication and trust.[39] When it comes to race, ethnicity, and culture, cultural humility needs to be part of self-reflection. Cultural humility is defined as "a process of reflection and lifelong inquiry, involves self-awareness of personal and cultural biases as well as awareness and sensitivity to significant cultural issues of others."[46] Cultural humility means not only learning about different cultures but also reflecting on one's own cultures and how they have influenced one's values, assumptions, and biases.

This awareness of how one's cultures influence day-to-day life can bring us better understanding of how other individuals may be influenced by theirs.

SETTING UP THE ENVIRONMENT: INSTITUTIONAL CULTURE

Before launching or updating an inclusive mentorship program or relationship, it is important to ensure an inclusive environment. This includes addressing inclusion, or lack thereof, in both culture and leadership, as well as a commitment to invest adequate and appropriate resources.[47] Inviting a person with a marginalized identity into an environment without inclusion can damage the relationship at its inception.

A study of environmental scientists showed that inclusion and team procedural justice were associated with fewer negative mentoring experiences and greater mentoring satisfaction. The association was even stronger for BIPOC mentees when compared with their white counterparts. When BIPOC mentees reported levels of inclusivity, mentorship satisfaction increased as inclusivity increased.[48]

Assessment of the current institutional culture is an important starting point. If one does not know where they are, they would not know how to move forward. The Association of American Veterinary Medical Colleges has published an Intentional Organizational Diversity & Inclusion Efforts Assessment Tool that can be used to aid in culture assessment.[49]

Climate surveys can also be used as an assessment tool. It is important to maintain confidentiality to get truthful responses on such surveys. Maintaining confidentiality can be a challenge in veterinary medicine, in particular, due to the significant lack or representation of BIPOC individuals in the field. If there are only one or two BIPOC individuals in a practice or workplace and race/ethnicity are tied to the survey responses, it can be challenging to prevent their survey responses from being tied to a specific person. However, it is critical to get the perspective of those with marginalized identities. It is important to center the experiences of those individuals who are most affected by lack of inclusion in their environments.[4] Hiring an independent diversity, equity, inclusion, and belonging (DEIB) consultant who can glean meaningful information from survey responses without tying responses to specific individuals may help overcome this barrier.

Ways to foster an inclusive climate include, but are not limited to

- Diversity of team composition[48,50]
- Focus on interpersonal skills, including social sensitivity and emotional engagement[48,50]
- Open participation in decision making[48,50]
- Creation and implementation of fair and transparent policies, for example, in authorship practices for publications[48,51]
- Consistent and equal application and enforcement of policies[48]
- Teamwork training and exercises[48,50]
- Ongoing professional development on mentorship and the aforementioned components[48]

PROGRAM DESIGN AND MATCHING

Mentorship program design should incorporate inclusion as a core tenant. Looking at each step in the process through the lens of inclusivity and critical mentorship can keep the focus on those individuals with marginalized identities who may need different kinds of resources and support. Critical mentorship incorporates awareness and acknowledgment of mentees' social identities and how they affect mentees' interactions and learning styles.

When designing or redesigning a mentorship program, it is important to remember that mentees and mentors do not need to share social identities to be successful. Veterinary medicine has significant underrepresentation in terms of race and ethnicity, meaning access to mentors who share their identity is more difficult for BIPOC than in other fields. Homophily, a tendency to associate and connect with those who share similarities,[52] plays a role in this lack of access. Although this is often an unintended barrier, acknowledging differences in social identity and associated privilege can help minimize homophily's influence on mentor/mentee selection and the mentoring relationship.

BIPOC and women mentees placed more value on being matched with mentors who shared their own race or gender and reported receiving more help. However, matching race and/or gender between mentors and mentees has not been shown to affect academic outcomes.[53] Sharing of similar attitudes between mentees and mentors has been shown to be more important to a successful mentoring relationship than sharing social identities.[27,54] Attitudinal similarities that increase mentee satisfaction include similarities in values, general outlook, and problem-solving approach.[54] Asking questions to explore these attitudes before entering a mentoring relationship can help mentees find a mentor they are more likely to connect with. Mentees with oppressed identities can, with the prospective mentor's consent, consider discussing specific areas related to their oppressed identities, such as systemic racism, cultural humility, discrimination, proactive pronoun use, privilege, implicit bias, and so on.

MENTOR TRAINING

Training of mentors before engaging in mentorship is critical to a successful relationship. Without adequate preparation, there is a risk of unsuccessful mentorship. Poor communication and mentor's lack of experience are commonly cited causes for failure of mentoring relationships.[40] Training on how negative mentoring experiences can harm relationships can bring awareness to the importance of fostering inclusion.[48]

Training on interpersonal skills and teamwork are important to inclusivity.[48,50] Training should also specifically include components on social identities like race, gender, sexuality, and class. When social identities and their impacts are not considered, there is a risk of alienating mentees with marginalized identities. Training should be culturally relevant so mentors can understand their mentee's cultural context as well as how their culture affects their values and perspectives.[4,47] It is also important to consider intersectional identities. The needs of black women can differ from the needs of black men, or BIPOC LGBTQIA+ youth. It is also important to recognize each person as an individual with their own individual perspectives as social identities are not monolithic.

Perceived lack of competence is a barrier to mentors initiating and facilitating discussions on DEIB topics with their mentees.[55] Training can mitigate this barrier. Some DEIB topics that are pertinent to mentorship include, but are not limited to:

- Inclusivity
- Equity
- Belonging
- Psychological safety
- Intersectionality
- Cultural humility
- Cultural responsiveness
- Microaggressions and macroaggressions

- Power dynamics
- Implicit bias
- Stereotype threat
- Identity cover

The lack of diversity in veterinary medicine involves barriers to the field that are faced by marginalized individuals and communities. Understanding these barriers and the challenges they present to BIPOC individuals entering and advancing in the veterinary field can help one identify the power dynamics at play both in the relationship and the profession.

Power dynamics are defined as "the ways power works in a setting"[56] and are important to consider in inclusive mentorship; this includes formal power that is derived from one's position or title and informal power that derives from one's influence over others.[56] Those with privileged identities hold informal power. Privilege is defined as "certain social advantages, benefits, or degrees of prestige and respect that an individual has by virtue of belonging to certain social identity groups."[57] Research suggests practices that incorporate navigating power differentials in the mentoring relationship, especially across race and gender, can reduce stereotype threat and increase feelings of belonging for individuals with marginalized identities.[41]

It is common to have power differential between mentors and mentees in traditional hierarchical mentorship, which can lead to mentees being vulnerable to exploitation.[24,58] There should be a discussion on power differentials early in the mentoring relationship and how to avoid their influence. In veterinary medicine, due to the lack of diversity in terms of race and ethnicity, individuals with privileged identities are more often in the position to mentor and hold more both formal and informal power in many mentoring relationships. Perceived power differentials can vary due to cultural influences, as well as on an individual level.[24] Cultural knowledge of one's mentee can help mentors recognize, acknowledge, and discuss these differentials more readily. It is important to remember that advice that has worked for a mentor with a privileged identity may not work in the same way for mentees with marginalized identities.

When there are power imbalances, trust can be more difficult to earn and easier to lose.[24] Mentoring relationships with a higher power differential result in decreased initiative, creativity, and empowerment of mentees.[41] When mentees perceive a larger power differential, they are often less comfortable initiating communication with their mentor.[24] Power dynamics have also been shown to affect closeness in mentoring relationships and subsequently associated social capital.[41] Power structures can affect accountability in mentoring relationships due to reticence to give critical and honest feedback as well as few consequences for negative mentoring experiences.[24] Strategies that can decrease power differentials in mentoring relationships include facilitated mentorship, choice, and collaborative peer mentorship.[58]

ONGOING ASSESSMENT AND MAINTENANCE

Fostering inclusivity is an ongoing process and requires maintenance. Complacency can risk damaging trust. Periodic evaluation is important to make sure the relationship is improving and meeting the needs of both the mentor and mentee. Open and honest feedback is critical to the mentoring relationship, and positive responses from mentors to feedback can increase trust.[24] Power dynamics can be a barrier to open feedback and should be considered when soliciting and receiving feedback.

Periodic reminders and training can keep inclusivity and belonging as priorities in mentoring relationships. Cultivating open communication, trust, psychological safety, cultural humility, and transparency requires continued focus and action throughout the relationship. Reminders to consider and discuss how privilege and power dynamics impact the relationship can help one navigate the ongoing impact they have on mentees, mentors, and the relationship.

SUMMARY

Inclusive mentorship has the potential to improve many aspects of the veterinary field, including lack of representation, providing exposure to multiple viewpoints, increasing feelings of belonging, decreasing burnout, and improving retention, among others. It is important to center the people who are most affected by a lack of inclusion when designing mentorship programs, namely, individuals who hold marginalized social identities, including people who are BIPOC, LGBTQIA+, women, disabled, and so on. Creating more inclusive environments and relationships directly benefits marginalized individuals, and also benefits those with privileged identities. Transparency, psychological safety, and good communication can be beneficial for any person in a mentorship program. Conversely, when the focus is on those who hold privileged identities, barriers will prevent full, authentic participation by those who hold oppressed identities. With the significant underrepresentation of BIPOC in veterinary medicine, a field with one of lowest rates of diversity in terms of race and ethnicity, it is especially important to center BIPOC people in our mentorship programs and relationships.

Veterinary medicine has a duty to support our ever-diversifying society. Mentorship plays a critical role in veterinary medicine, and a commitment to inclusion within our mentorship programs and relationships sets the stage to improve ourselves and the profession throughout our careers. Inclusion in mentorship and throughout the field provides us the opportunity to strengthen our profession, our bonds with each other, and our ability to serve our patients and our clients.

CLINICS CARE POINTS

- Critical mentorship incorporates the context of the social identities of mentors and mentees in the design and functioning of the mentoring relationship.
- Mentorship that is not inclusive can have a detrimental effect on people with marginalized identities. This can lead to a negative view of the profession at large and higher rates of attrition.
- Mentors who feel they lack competence in DEIB topics with their mentees are less likely to initiate and facilitate discussions on DEIB topics.

DISCLOSURE

The author has no conflicts of interest to disclose.

REFERENCES

1. U.S. Bureau of Labor Statistics. Employed persons by detailed occupation, sex, race, and Hispanic or Latino ethnicity. BLS.gov. 2024. Available at: https://www. bls.gov/cps/cpsaat11.htm. Accessed February 5, 2024.
2. Henry-Noel N, Bishop M, Gwede CK, et al. Mentorship in medicine and other health professions. J Cancer Educ 2019;34(4):629–37.

3. World Bank. 2013. Inclusion Matters: The Foundation for Shared Prosperity. Washington, DC: World Bank. License: Creative Commons Attribution CC BY 3.0. https://doi.org/10.1596/978-1-4648-0010-8.

4. Weiston T. How to "do" critical mentoring: making your program more culturally relevant. The Chronicle of Evidence-Based Mentoring. 2018. Available at: https://www.evidencebasedmentoring.org/how-to-do-critical-mentoring-making-your-program-more-culturally-relevant/#_ftn1. Accessed February 5, 2024.

5. Mor Barak ME, Levin A. Outside of the corporate mainstream and excluded from the work community: A study of diversity, job satisfaction and well-being. Community Work Fam 2002;5(2):133–57.

6. Wallace JE. Meaningful work and well-being: a study of the positive side of veterinary work. Vet Rec 2019;185(18):571.

7. Hagerty BM, Lynch-Sauer J, Patusky KL, et al. Sense of belonging: a vital mental health concept. Arch Psychiatr Nurs 1992 Jun;6(3):172–7.

8. van der Velden GJ, Meeuwsen JA, Fox CM, et al. Peer-mentorship and first-year inclusion: building belonging in higher education. BMC Med Educ 2023;23(000).

9. Wright-Mair R. Longing to belong: mentoring relationships as a pathway to fostering a sense of belonging for racially minoritized faculty at predominantly white institutions. Journal Committed to Social Change on Race and Ethnicity (JCSCORE) 2020;6(2):2–31.

10. Haeger H, Fresquez C. Mentoring for inclusion: the impact of mentoring on undergraduate researchers in the sciences. CBE-Life Sci Educ 2016;15(3):ar36.

11. Master A, Meltzoff AN. Cultural stereotypes and sense of belonging contribute to gender gaps in STEM. International Journal of Gender, Science and Technology 2020;12(1):152–98.

12. Thoman DB, Smith JL, Brown ER, et al. Beyond performance: a motivational experiences model of stereotype threat. Educ Psychol Rev 2013;25:211–43.

13. Mello ZR, Mallett RK, Andretta JR, et al. Stereotype threat and school belonging in adolescents from diverse racial/ethnic backgrounds. J Risk Issues 2012; 17(1):9–14.

14. Steele CM, Aronson J. Stereotype threat and the intellectual test performance of African Americans. J Pers Soc Psychol 1995;69(5):797–811.

15. Logel C, Walton GM, Spencer SJ, et al. Interacting with sexist men triggers social identity threat among female engineers [published correction appears in J Pers Soc Psychol. 2009 Oct,97(4).578]. J Pers Soc Psychol 2009;96(6).1089–103.

16. Holleran SE, Whitehead J, Schmader T, et al. Talking shop and shooting the breeze: a study of workplace conversation and job disengagement among STEM faculty. Soc Psychol Personal Sci 2011;2(1):65–71.

17. Volk J, Schimmack U, Strand E, et al. Merck animal health veterinary wellbeing study III. Merck Animal Health 2022. Available at: https://www.merck-animal-health-usa.com/about-us/veterinary-wellbeing-study. Accessed February 11, 2024.

18. Jordan J, Watcha D, Cassella C, et al. Impact of a mentorship program on medical student burnout. AEM Educ Train 2019;3(3):218–25. Published 2019 May 23.

19. Cavanaugh K, Cline D, Belfer B, et al. The positive impact of mentoring on burnout: Organizational research and best practices. Journal of Interprofessional Education & Practice 2022;28:100521.

20. Walker VP, Williams DR. Restitution through equity-focused mentoring: a solution to diversify the physician workforce. Front Public Health 2022;10:879181. Published 2022 Jun 1.

21. Friedman DB, Yelton B, Corwin SJ, et al. Value of peer mentorship for equity in higher education leadership: A school of public health focus with implications for all academic administrators. Mentor Tutoring: Partnership in Learning 2021; 29(5):500–21.

22. Lan YL, Huang WT, Kao CL, et al. The relationship between organizational climate, job stress, workplace burnout, and retention of pharmacists. J Occup Health 2020;62(1):e12079.

23. Brook J, Aitken LM, MacLaren JA, et al. An intervention to decrease burnout and increase retention of early career nurses: a mixed methods study of acceptability and feasibility. BMC Nurs 2021;20(19).

24. Hund AK, Churchill AC, Faist AM, et al. Transforming mentorship in STEM by training scientists to be better leaders. Ecol Evol 2018;8(20):9962–74. Published 2018 Oct 2.

25. Reinhard AR, Hains KD, Hains BJ, et al. Are they ready? Trials, tribulations, and professional skills vital for new veterinary graduate success. Front Vet Sci 2021;8: 785844.

26. British Veterinary Association. BVA report on discrimination in the veterinary profession. British Veterinary Association; 2019. Available at: https://www.bva.co.uk/media/2991/bva-report-on-discrimination-in-the-veterinary-profession.pdf. Accessed February 11, 2024.

27. Geraci SA, Thigpen SC. A review of mentoring in academic medicine. Am J Med Sci 2017;353(2):151–7.

28. Brown BP, Zablah AR, Bellenger DN. The role of mentoring in promoting organizational commitment among black managers: An evaluation of the indirect effects of racial similarity and shared racial perspectives. J Bus Res 2008;61:732–8.

29. Page SE. The diversity bonus: how great teams pay off in the knowledge economy. Princeton: Princeton University Press; 2017.

30. Efstathiou JA, Drumm MR, Paly JP, et al. Long-term impact of a faculty mentoring program in academic medicine. PLoS One 2018;13(11):e0207634.

31. Sue DW, Capodilupo CM, Torino GC, et al. Racial microaggressions in everyday life: implications for clinical practice. Am Psychol 2007;62(4):271–86.

32. Anderson N, Lett E, Asabor EN, et al. The association of microaggressions with depressive symptoms and institutional satisfaction among a national cohort of medical students. J Gen Intern Med 2022;37(2):298–307.

33. Mizrahi I. The minority-majority shift: two decades that will change america—for the health and wellness industry, it's time for a check-up. Forbes 2022. Available at: https://www.forbes.com/sites/isaacmizrahi/2020/04/29/the-minority-majority-shift-two-decades-that-will-change-america-for-the-health–wellness-industry-its-time-for-a-check-up/?sh=517d1b4246ce. Accessed February 20, 2024.

34. Lu D, Smart C, Gamio L. Where the Racial Makeup of the U.S. Shifted in the Last Decade. N Y Times 2021. Available at: https://www.nytimes.com/interactive/2021/08/12/us/2020-census-race-ethnicity.html. Accessed February 20, 2024.

35. American Veterinary Medical Association. AVMA pet ownership and demographics sourcebook 2018.

36. Park RM, Gruen ME, Royal K. Association between dog owner demographics and decision to seek veterinary care. Veterinary Sciences 2021;8(1):7.

37. Decker Sparks JL, Camacho B, Tedeschi P, et al. Race and ethnicity are not primary determinants in utilizing veterinary services in underserved communities in the United States. J Appl Anim Welfare Sci 2018;21(2):120–9.

38. Gandenberger J, Hawes SM, Wheatall E, et al. Development and initial validation of the Animal Welfare Cultural Competence Inventory (AWCCI) to assess cultural competence in animal welfare. J Appl Anim Welfare Sci 2023;26(4):540–51.

39. Fleseriu M, Lim DST. Mentorship in academic medicine: truth is in the eye of the beholder. Nat Rev Endocrinol 2023;19(7):373–4.

40. Straus SE, Johnson MO, Marquez C, et al. Characteristics of successful and failed mentoring relationships: a qualitative study across two academic health centers. Acad Med 2013;88(1):82–9.

41. National Academies of Sciences. Engineering, and Medicine; Policy and Global Affairs; Board on Higher Education and Workforce; Committee on Effective Mentoring in STEMM. Science of Mentoring Relationships: What Is Mentorship?. In: Dahlberg ML, Byars-Winston A, editors. The science of effective mentorship in STEMM. Washington (DC): National Academies Press (US); 2019. Available at: https://www.ncbi.nlm.nih.gov/books/NBK552775/.

42. Edmondson A. Psychological safety and learning behavior in work teams. Adm Sci Q 1999;44(2):350–83.

43. Tsuei SH, Lee D, Ho C, Regehr G, Nimmon I . Exploring the Construct of Psychological Safety in Medical Education. Acad Med. 2019;94(11S Association of American Medical Colleges Learn Serve Lead: Proceedings of the 58th Annual Research in Medical Education Sessions):S28-S35.

44. Campeau M. Beyond diversity] uncovering talent: a conversation with Kenji Yoshino. HR Professional Now; 2018. Available at: http://hrprofessionalnow.ca/latest-news/526-beyond-diversity-uncovering-talent-a-conversation-with-kenji-yoshino. Accessed March 8, 2024.

45. Deloitte. Uncovering talent: A new model of inclusion. 2019. Available at: https://www2.deloitte.com/content/dam/Deloitte/us/Documents/about-deloitte/us-about-deloitte-uncovering-talent-a-new-model-of-inclusion.pdf. Accessed March 8, 2024.

46. Yeager KA, Bauer-Wu S. Cultural humility: essential foundation for clinical researchers. Appl Nurs Res 2013;26(4):251–6.

47. Azevedo L, Haupt B, Shi W. Equitable and inclusive mentoring programs for women faculty. J Publ Aff Educ 2023;29(4):441–61.

48. Robotham KJ, Settles IH, Spence Cheruvelil K, et al. Just and inclusive team climates affect mentoring satisfaction: the roles of negative mentoring and race. J Career Dev 2022;49(6):1367–85.

49. Association of American Veterinary Medical Colleges. Intentional Organizational Diversity & Inclusion Efforts Assessment Tool. 2020. Available at: https://www.aavmc.org/assets/Site_18/files/Diversity/AAVMC-Organizational%20Diversity.Inclusion%20Assessment%20-%20June%202020.pdf. Accessed March 10, 2024.

50. Cheruvelil KS, Soranno PA, Weathers KC, et al. Creating and maintaining high-performing collaborative research teams: the importance of diversity and interpersonal skills. Front Ecol Environ 2014;12(1):31–8.

51. Oliver SK, Fergus CE, Skaff NK, et al. Strategies for effective collaborative manuscript development in interdisciplinary science teams. Innovative Viewpoints 2018;9(4):e02206.

52. McPherson M, Smith-Lovin L, Cook JM. Birds of a feather: homophily in social networks. Ann Rev Sociol 2001;27(1):415–44.

53. Blake-Beard S, Bayne ML, Crosby FJ, et al. Matching by race and gender in mentoring relationships: keeping our eyes on the prize. J Soc Issues 2011;67(3):622–43.

54. Ensher EA, Grant-Vallone EJ, Marelich WD. Effects of perceived attitudinal and demographic similarity on protégés' support and satisfaction gained from their mentoring relationships. J Appl Soc Psychol 2002;32(7):1407–30.

55. Chao D, Badwan M, Briceño EM. ADDRESSING diversity, equity, inclusion and belonging (DEIB) in mentorship relationships. J Clin Exp Neuropsychol 2022; 44(5–6):420–40.

56. Bates K, Silva Parker C, Ogden C. Power dynamics: the hidden element to effective meetings. Interaction Institute for Social Change 2018. Available at: https://interactioninstitute.org/power-dynamics-the-hidden-element-to-effective-meetings. Accessed March 14, 2024.

57. Rider University. Privilege and intersectionality. University Libraries at Rider University; 2023. Available at: https://guides.rider.edu/privilege. Accessed March 19, 2024.

58. Cross M, Lee S, Bridgman H, et al. Benefits, barriers and enablers of mentoring female health academics: An integrative review. PLoS One 2019;14(4):e0215319.

Caring for the Caregivers
Supporting the Mental Health & Wellbeing of a Diverse Veterinary Team

Angie Arora, MSW, RSW*

KEYWORDS

• Veterinary mental health • Veterinary wellbeing • Trauma • Compassion fatigue

KEY POINTS

- Professional quality of life must be understood from an equitable and inclusive lens to be applicable to the diverse realities of veterinary professionals.
- Oppression needs to be understood as a form of trauma.
- Any efforts veterinary medicine makes to address the mental health and wellbeing of its people must consider barriers to access for diverse communities.

INTRODUCTION

Veterinary medicine operates as a microcosm of broader society, and the issues impacting the world at large impact the people of the profession. Two issues for which this is the case are mental health and diversity, equity, inclusion, and belonging.

With growing attention to issues of mental health and wellbeing, veterinary medicine has embarked on its own journey of understanding factors impacting the psychological, emotional, physical, and social health of its people. However, 1 often overlooked nuance is how the health of diverse professionals is differentially impacted by the lack of diversity, equity, inclusion, and belonging in veterinary medicine. Herein lies the missing link: discussions of diversity, equity, inclusion, and belonging must address wellbeing; discussions of wellbeing must address diversity, equity, inclusion, and belonging. For far too long, the profession and the world at large have failed to draw a direct correlation between the two. The purpose of this article is to shed light onto the inextricable link between the two so that no one is left behind as the health of the profession and its people advance.

PROFESSIONAL QUALITY OF LIFE

The mental health and wellbeing of veterinary professionals is impacted by several factors including personal upbringing, exposure to stress and trauma, learning

Arora Wellness, Ontario, Canada
* Arora Wellness, 1108-250 Consumers Road, #774, North York, Ontario M2V 4V6, Canada.
E-mail address: angie@angiearora.com

Vet Clin Small Anim 54 (2024) 881–888
https://doi.org/10.1016/j.cvsm.2024.07.015   **vetsmall.theclinics.com**

environments, and workplace conditions. In all these factors, more nuanced experiences of discrimination and oppression are often present, differentially impacting marginalized groups of professionals. Understanding how these nuanced experiences connect to professional quality of life is critical to ensuring responses to veterinary mental health are equitable and inclusive.

Professional quality of life refers to the positive and challenging aspects a person experiences in relation to his or her work and is experienced as either compassion fatigue or compassion satisfaction.[1] While compassion satisfaction refers to deriving pleasure and fulfillment from one's helping work, compassion fatigue refers to the cumulative experience of unresolved exposure to burnout and secondary traumatic stress (**Fig. 1**).

The following section will provide a deeper analysis into the importance of understanding burnout, trauma, and compassion fatigue from an equitable and inclusive lens.

Burnout

Burnout is widely understood as the cumulative impact of exposure to chronic stress that remains unaddressed and unmanaged, leading to a host of psychological, emotional, physical, social, and spiritual impacts. According to the Areas of Worklife Model,[2] the 6 key causes of burnout at work include

- Workload: Insufficient time and support to fully recover from demanding work creates vulnerability to chronic exhaustion. Exposure to emotionally taxing situations like those present in veterinary medicine further exacerbates this vulnerability.
- Control: The perceived or actual lack of control over one's work can present as role ambiguity (the absence of clarity or direction in one's work) and lack of autonomy, both which contribute to people's experiences of stress at work.
- Reward: Insufficient financial, verbal, and social rewards from the workplace can increase team members' vulnerability to burnout. However, when one experiences excessive rewards, those who do not may perceive themselves as contributing less, which can also create conditions of stress.
- Values: The extent to which a person can work in accordance with his or her ideals, motivations, and values can contribute to experiences of burnout. When there is an alignment between organizational and personal values (value

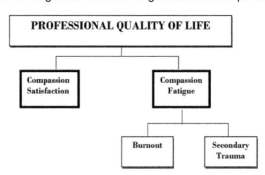

Fig. 1. A comparative analysis of burnout and professional quality of life in clinical mental health providers and health care administrators–scientific figure on ResearchGate. (Newell, J. M., & MacNeil, G. A. (2011). A Comparative Analysis of Burnout and Professional Quality of Life in Clinical Mental Health Providers and Health Care Administrators. Journal of Workplace Behavioral Health, 26(1), 25-43. https://doi.org/10.1080/15555240.2011.540978. & Stamm, B. H. (2008). The ProQOL. Available at www.proqol.org.)

congruence), team members' capacity to thrive flourishes; however, when there is a lack of alignment, they are more susceptible to burnout.

- Fairness: When rewards, opportunities, and recognition are experienced fairly across the organization, this creates feelings of mutual trust and collaboration. Fair decisions are ones that consider the diverse conditions and realities of its team members. When this fairness lacks, team members are less likely to accept organizational change and are more susceptible to burnout.
- Community: The social support one receives from supervisors, colleagues, and family members can act as buffers to burnout, suggesting that the quality of human interactions directly correlates with how people relate to their work.

Conceptualizing burnout this way suggests that the impacts of chronic stress are not simply caused by a lack of personal willpower or insufficient coping mechanisms, but rather are deeply impacted by systemic policies, practices, and norms.

Mainstream understanding of professional burnout does not often view these root causes from the perspective of diversity, equity, inclusion, and belonging. Doing so helps one understand that burnout impacts people differently depending on their social identity and exposure to discrimination and oppression.

Take for example, the root cause of fairness. Veterinary professionals who experience microaggressions, lack of equitable access to promotions, or direct exposure to discrimination from clients or colleagues will have experienced a lack of fairness yet may not consciously attribute this to their overall experience of burnout. Not seeing oneself represented in the workplace (eg, gender identity, age, race, culture, ethnicity, ability) may subconsciously impact the professional's ability to feel a sense of community, thereby impacting his or her sense of belonging within the team.

Without conceptualizing burnout from this equitable and inclusive lens, mainstream wellness strategies and initiatives ignore the realities of diverse groups, thereby failing to the meet the needs of all people.

Trauma

Veterinary medicine is a profession that is highly exposed to stress and trauma. Although stress can be best understood as a natural human response to challenging situations,[3] trauma is better understood as a highly personalized response to something that overwhelms one's capacity to cope, because the situation causing the trauma is out of the ordinary.[4] Whereas most experiences of trauma are stressful, not all experiences of stress are traumatic.

Veterinary medicine is only beginning to appreciate its high exposure to trauma, be it the treatment of animals or the exposure to clients' and colleagues' pain and suffering. Even less understood is how the exposure to discrimination and oppression may also result in trauma. More recent studies are beginning to draw a direct correlation between oppression and mental wellbeing including psychological distress and suicide ideation. For example, 1 study conducted by Scoresby and colleagues found that experiences of sexism, classism, ageism, and ableism were strong predictors of psychological distress in veterinary professionals.[5]

The oppressive experiences of marginalized communities are often not labeled or understood as traumatic. Because trauma is often understood as an acute experience that overwhelms one's capacity to cope, the insidious, historical, and collective nature of sexism, racism, ableism, classism, and heterosexism are not often perceived as directly harmful to one's health and wellbeing. "When discriminatory experiences are superimposed on a backdrop of trauma, individuals may be more likely to suffer psychological distress."[6] Therefore, when understanding the trauma of people belonging to socially oppressed groups, the acute experiences of pain (eg, microaggressions, harassment, bullying, and violence) must be understood just as deeply as collective experiences of pain (eg, historical oppression, social exclusion, and systemic barriers).

Failure to understand and acknowledge this connection prevents healing at individual and systemic levels. The victimization of those who have experienced oppression is often denied. Veterinary medicine is no exception. It has only been since 2020 where the pervasiveness of anti-Black racism reached peaked heights of discussion that the profession began to openly discuss its lack of diversity, equity, and inclusion, albeit with a high degree of resistance from some within the profession. These conversations have opened space to include more intersectional identities and experiences including but not limited to colonialism, ableism, and heterosexism.

Those who experience marginalization and oppression often subconsciously deny their own needs to survive, especially surviving in a system that is not representative of their social identities and unresponsive to their needs. This survival is best understood as living in chronic stress, and chronic states of nervous system dysregulation.

Compassion Fatigue

When exposure to burnout and trauma remain unaddressed and unresolved, professionals are at a higher risk for experiencing compassion fatigue, that is "the deep physical, emotional, and spiritual exhaustion that can result from working day to day in an intense caregiving environment."[7]

Without an understanding that discrimination and oppression contribute to the experience of burnout, trauma, and compassion fatigue, analysis remains limited and excludes the realities of those impacted by oppression based on race, culture, ethnicity, gender, gender identity and expression, sexual identity, ability, age, socioeconomic status, nationality, immigration status, and neurodiverse identities.

IMPACTS OF OPPRESSION ON VETERINARY HEALTH AND WELLBEING

It is now understood that life stressors can compromise people's mental health and wellbeing, and social groups more exposed to discrimination and oppression may experience particularly marked consequences.[6] Therefore, given the nuanced context of burnout, trauma, and compassion fatigue, understanding its impacts on diverse veterinary professionals is the next step to ensuring more equitable and inclusive forms of care.

Minority Stress Theory

Repeated, chronic, and unresolved exposure to trauma can overwhelm a person's ability to cope, which is better understood through the minority stress theory.[8] This theory suggests that the chronic exposure to inequities and disadvantages may lead to an accelerated decline in one's mental and physical health. This is not to suggest that unresolved stress and trauma do not impact all people, but rather, the additive stressors impacting marginalized communities create additional health challenges to navigate.

Living with a social identity that is predisposed to overt and covert harm causes one to learn to live on guard. This is experienced through increased vigilance and the anticipation of social rejection. Although often happening subconsciously, "the persistent use of 'high-effort coping' to combat acute and chronic stressors has disproportionate effects"[8] on the health of diverse communities leading to poorer health outcomes including accelerated aging and the degradation of key brain circuits involved in regulating emotions and cognition.[9]

Psychological safety

When people live on guard, it can be even more challenging to experience psychological safety at workplaces, which are often microcosms of the discrimination and oppression people are exposed to outside of work. According to Amy Edmondson, psychological safety can be understood as "the belief that one will not be punished or humiliated for speaking up with ideas, questions, concerns, or mistakes, and that the team is safe for interpersonal risk taking."[10]

Timothy R. Clark[11] provides a useful way of understanding psychological safety in the workplace through 4 stages.

1. Inclusion safety: Team members feel as though they belong at work, which is represented by feeling wanted and appreciated.
2. Learner safety: Team members feel safe enough to ask questions and admit mistakes without the fear of judgment or reprimand
3. Contributor safety: Team members feel safe enough to share their ideas without the fear of embarrassment or ridicule.
4. Challenger safety: Team members feel safe enough to question others' ideas and suggest changes to ideas, plans, and ways of working.

When viewed without an equitable and inclusive lens, one will fail to see how psychological safety can be experienced differently by diverse groups at work. For example, according to the American Veterinary Medical Association, 91% of veterinarians in 2022 were White; 4.4% were Asian, and 2.2% were Black.[12] It is difficult to experience a full sense of belonging when one does not see his or her identity reflected in the people with whom he or she works. For those who are used to not seeing their identities and experiences reflected in those around them, it is common for the nervous system to subconsciously scan the room for cues of safety. This feeling of not belonging is reinforced by microaggressions, colloquial Eurocentric language and jokes, tokenism, and overt discrimination.

When microaggressions and overt discrimination do occur in the workplace, the inability of team members, management, and leadership to address such harm will only further exacerbate the lack of safety those from under-represented communities feel. According to a study by the Ontario Veterinary Medical Association, 59% of its survey respondents said they have witnessed discriminatory behaviors in veterinary medicine, but only 30% felt confident that action would be taken to address the harm.[13] Here one sees that the failure to build on the 4 stages of psychological safety can lead to a deep sense of distrust and apathy in the workplace and the profession at large.

Resilience

When exploring the challenges of diverse social groups, it is equally important to understand how communities have learned to cope despite oppressive systems and structures. This is often referred to as resilience, that is, the "process and outcome of adapting to difficult or challenging life experiences, especially through mental, emotional, and behavioral flexibility and adjustment for external and internal demands."[14]

There is a rightful resistance to oppressed communities needing to be resilient, because it places an undo responsibility on those who have been harmed to cope with systems that have the responsibility to change. However, the mental health and wellbeing of marginalized communities cannot wait for systems to change, and ensuring adequate self and community care is essential to surviving and thriving.

CULTIVATING INCLUSIVE VETERINARY WELLBEING

With this increased understanding of how diverse veterinary professionals may experience additive stressors impacting their mental health and wellbeing comes a responsibility to cultivate more equitable and inclusive professional wellbeing. Any efforts to adequately address the lack of diversity in veterinary medicine and promote more equitable and inclusive workplaces will have a positive impact on the mental health and wellbeing of its people. Any efforts to ensure mental health and wellbeing initiatives adequately factor in the realities of diverse lived experiences will also have a positive impact on mental health and wellbeing.

The following section provides considerations for veterinary professionals and hospitals that may lead to more equitable and inclusive wellbeing support.

Reducing Barriers to Self-Care

Traditional understanding of self-care is the "individual or professional pursuit for stress reduction at a physical, psychological, and emotional level to minimize compassion fatigue, enhance personal wellbeing, and manage exposure to trauma."[15] This holds value for all veterinary professionals when recovering from the frequent exposure to stress and trauma in veterinary medicine. For those who experience a disproportionate exposure to trauma because of discrimination and oppression, these coping strategies become imperative for survival.

However, mainstream wellness practices are often riddled with cultural appropriation. "When a dominant culture takes from another culture–usually a minority or disadvantaged culture–without the full regard for the context, respect or reverence, or even acknowledgment of the culture it's taking from, it is cultural appropriation."[16] When mainstream methods of self-care such as breathwork, yoga, and mindfulness are offered without an equitable and inclusive lens, some people may not feel safe to access them, especially when their cultural practices are being co-opted for a fad or commodification.

Furthermore, it is crucial that wellness practitioners invited into veterinary medicine spaces are consciously reducing barriers to access. Does the wellness practitioner understand and avoid cultural appropriation? Are neurodivergent needs considered and safe options presented? Does the wellness practitioner consider a range of physical abilities and accommodate accordingly? Does the wellness practitioner understand how historical, collective, and insidious oppression impact acute trauma for diverse groups in the profession?

Re-envisioning Self-Care

For veterinary professionals who have experienced microagressions, discrimination, and overt and covert oppression within and outside the profession, self-care takes on a new meaning. In a world where one has subconsciously learned to survive, finding ways to restore and heal is imperative for an enhanced state of wellbeing.

Professionals should consider several things:

- Because stress and unresolved exposure to trauma live in the body, learning about one's nervous system can be an empowering way to understand one's coping strategies and behaviors. This, followed by learning how to regulate one's nervous system is a powerful way of reclaiming power.

- Seek mental health professionals who embody antioppressive and trauma-informed principles into their practice to better ensure one's lived realities are understood in the context of systemic oppression.
- Form meaningful bonds with others who understand one's lived experiences by creating community networks. This can help to improve one's sense of validation and positive self-concept, leading to improved feelings of belonging.
- Become involved with affinity and advocacy groups working to promote more equitable and inclusive veterinary medicine. This communal expression of advocacy can provide emotional and psychological relief, reducing feelings of isolation and helplessness.

Embracing Collective Care

The Western way of individual living runs counter to the collective way of living many around the world are accustomed to. "The emphasis on the interconnectedness between individual healing and broader community healing has been critical in the history of various activism movements, including, Indigenous activism, peer-based recovery communities, 2SLGBTTQIA + TQIA+ and queer liberation movements, HIV/AIDS movements, disability justice collectives, Black liberation movements, and women's health movements."[15] Despite this, mainstream wellness discourse has prioritized individual self-care over collective care.

Veterinary medicine can counter this narrative by

- Continuing to support peer-based mentorship programming that fosters community growth and healing
- Intentionally seeking mental health professionals from diverse communities (who may be outside of the profession), who are more representative of diverse social identities and practice with informed understandings of historical and collective oppression
- Integrating veterinary social workers from diverse social groups who can support employee mental health and wellbeing.
- Creating structured, consistent practices within the hospital that foster team-level discussions such as debriefing
- Develop and facilitate employee resource groups (internal communities of workers with shared identities and interests[17]) as a way of cultivating safer spaces for those who may feel excluded and lack psychological safety in the workplace
- Encouraging professionals to participate in affinity and advocacy-based organizations as a way of fostering community connection and systemic change

SUMMARY

While there are many factors impacting the mental health and wellbeing of veterinary professionals, experiencing discrimination and oppression is one that can no longer be ignored. Because it contributes to the nuanced experience of burnout, trauma, and compassion fatigue, diverse veterinary professionals are experiencing negative impacts on their health and relationships within the workplace. Veterinary medicine has a responsibility to reduce barriers to equitable support and improve the nature of collective healing so all its people can thrive in the work they love.

DISCLOSURE

The author has nothing to disclose.

REFERENCES

1. Tran ANP, To QG, Huynh VN, et al. Professional quality of life and its associated factors among Vietnamese doctors and nurses. BMC Health Serv Res 2023; 23(1):924. PMID: 37649084; PMCID: PMC10469419.
2. Leiter MP, Maslach C. Six areas of worklife: a model of the organizational context of burnout. J Health Hum Serv Adm 1999;21(4):472–89.
3. World Health Organization, Stress, Available at: https://www.who.int/news-room/questions-and-answers/item/stress. (Accessed March 1 2024), 2023.
4. Psychology Today, Trauma | Psychology Today. Psychology Today, Available at: https://www.psychologytoday.com/us/basics/trauma. (Accessed February 15 2024), 2019.
5. Scoresby K, Jurney C, Fackler A, et al. Relationships between diversity demographics, psychological distress, and suicidal thinking in the veterinary profession: a nationwide cross-sectional study during COVID-19. Front Vet Sci 2023; 10. https://doi.org/10.3389/fvets.2023.1130826.
6. Matheson K, Foster MD, Bombay A, et al. Traumatic experiences, perceived discrimination, and psychological distress among members of various socially marginalized groups. Front Psychol 2019;10:416.
7. Figley CR, Roop RG. Compassion fatigue in the animal-care community. Washington DC: Humane Society Press; 2006.
8. Hobson JM, Moody MD, Sorge RE, et al. The neurobiology of social stress resulting from racism: implications for pain disparities among racialized minorities. Neurobiol Pain 2022;12:100101.
9. Sima R. Racism takes a toll on the brain, research shows. Wash Post. 2023, Available at: https://www.washingtonpost.com/wellness/2023/02/16/racism-brain-mental-health-impact/. (Accessed February 15 2024).
10. What is Psychological Safety? – Psychological Safety, Available at: https://psychsafety.co.uk/about-psychological-safety/. (Accessed March 25 2024).
11. AVMA, AVMA Report on the Economic State of the Veterinary Profession. Available at: https://ebusiness.avma.org/files/ProductDownloads/eco-state-of-profession-report-lr-secured-2022.pdf, (Accessed February 15 2024), 2022.
12. OVMA. Building equity, diversity and inclusion in the profession. OVMA Focus Magazine 2023;42(1):18.
13. Clark TR. The 4 stages of psychological safety: defining the path to inclusion and innovation. Oakland, CA: Berrett-Koehler Publishers; 2020.
14. American Psychological Association. Resilience. American Psychological Association, Available at: https://www.apa.org/topics/resilience, (Accessed March 1 2024), 2022.
15. Bridging self-care and community care: integrated practices of student wellness and resilience, Available at: https://static1.squarespace.com/static/5aa5ba6e4611a06cb715dcf6/t/6115a4ae5fbcd069c8629b23/1628808378067/05-2101_BridgingSelfCare_Report_7.pdf, (Accessed March 24 2024), 2021.
16. How we can work together to avoid cultural appropriation in yoga. yogainternational.com, Available at: https://yogainternational.com/article/view/how-we-can-work-together-to-avoid-cultural-appropriation-in-yoga/. (Accessed January 23 2024).
17. Catalino N, Gardner N, Goldstein D, et al. Effective employee resource groups are key to inclusion at work. Here's how to get them right | McKinsey, Available at: https://www.mckinsey.com/capabilities/people-and-organizational-performance/our-insights/effective-employee-resource-groups-are-key-to-inclusion-at-work-heres-how-to-get-them-right, (Accessed February 15 2024), 2022.

Culturally Responsive Care in Veterinary Medicine

Sohaila Jafarian, DVM, MPH*

KEYWORDS

- Culturally responsive care • Aesculapian authority • Historical mistrust
- Demographics of pet owners • Human-animal bond • Veterinarians as caregivers
- Components of culturally responsive care

KEY POINTS

- Emphasizes the importance of understanding and addressing diverse cultural needs in veterinary practice to improve patient care and owner satisfaction.
- Discusses the historical influence of medical authority and its impact on trust, particularly through past abuses, shaping current perceptions and interactions in veterinary settings.
- Analyzes how the human-animal bond is consistent across various demographics, debunking common stereotypes about pet care preferences among different races, ethnicities, and income levels.
- Outlines the components of culturally responsive care, noting the scarcity of research in veterinary settings and drawing extensively from the substantial body of research in human medicine, especially nursing.
- Advocates for the integration of culturally responsive practices into veterinary care to address and overcome systemic barriers and enhance care for all clients. Discusses extrapolations from nursing literature regarding the consequences of inadequate culturally responsive care and the advantages of implementing such care.

INTRODUCTION

This article is an essential exploration of how veterinary medicine can better serve an increasingly diverse society through culturally responsive care. This article focuses on the interpersonal relationships between veterinarians, their teams, and pet owners, emphasizing the dynamics that influence trust and understanding in these interactions.

Transitioning from historical context to contemporary implications, this article redefines the role of veterinarians not only as providers of medical expertise but also as trusted caregivers. We then delve into what culturally responsive care entails within veterinary medicine, outlining its core components. This section also addresses the

* PO Box 1742, Silverdale, WA 98383.
E-mail address: JafarianDVM@gmail.com

Vet Clin Small Anim 54 (2024) 889–910
https://doi.org/10.1016/j.cvsm.2024.08.001
0195-5616/24/© 2024 Elsevier Inc. All rights reserved, including those for text and data mining, AI training, and similar technologies.
vetsmall.theclinics.com

profound implications of inadequate culturally responsive care, emphasizing the urgent need for a more inclusive and empathetic approach to veterinary service.

Further, we highlight the tangible benefits of implementing culturally responsive care. Such practices are shown to not only improve outcomes for animals and their owners but also to enhance the professional fulfillment and ethical standing of veterinarians. This underscores the dual benefits of culturally responsive care—improving patient outcomes while enriching the professional lives of veterinarians.

It is important to clarify that this article will not cover the spectrum of care, which involves the wide range of medical care options that veterinarians can provide. Instead, the focus of this article is on the critical interpersonal aspects of veterinary practice.

Ultimately, the aim of this article is to inspire a more empathetic, informed, and culturally competent veterinary community. By fostering respect, understanding, and humility, veterinarians are better equipped to meet the needs of all clients, thereby enhancing the overall efficacy and compassion of the veterinary field.

THE EVOLUTION OF AESCULAPIAN AUTHORITY IN VETERINARY PRACTICE

The concept of Aesculapian authority, a term derived from the ancient Roman "god of medicine" Aesculapius who was revered for his control over health and life, was traditionally reserved for the patient-physician relationship. This authority, as described by Kalisch in 1975, combines 3 distinct types of power. First is expert authority, whereby physicians, due to their extensive training, hold a monopoly on medical knowledge, traditionally leaving no room for patient rights or participation in medical decisions. This was based on the assumption that laypeople could not understand medical information and would likely harm themselves if they tried. Second, moral authority emerges from the physician's commitment to the Hippocratic oath, asserting a duty to always act in the patient's best interests, which historically translated into a controlling relationship over the patient. The third type is "God-given" authority, rooted in the physician's ability to navigate the mysteries of life and death, wielding the power to alleviate suffering and postpone the inevitable, thus commanding deep reverence and trust.[1] Supporting Kalisch's conclusions of the power of Aesculapian authority, Siegler and Osmond in their textbook Models of Madness, Models of Medicine,[2] argue that Aesculapian authority is far and away the most powerful authority in society as even kings, politicians, and dictators submit to medical authority they do not understand and can be ordered about by physicians.

Kalisch, drawing from her experiences as both a nurse and a patient, critiqued the traditional dynamics of this relationship between patient and physician, highlighting how patients often relinquish their autonomy, adopting a "sick role" that may strip them of dignity and resulting in distress and embarrassment. She pointed out that until the mid-twentieth century, such dynamics often operated without informed consent, leaving patients vulnerable to authoritarian medical practices. However, advancements such as the patient bill of rights and informed consent have begun to shift the relationship toward a more collaborative model, emphasizing shared decision-making and education.

Davis, a researcher who studied factors related to patient noncompliance, reported that a physician's attitude related to controlling the patient was influential in noncompliance.[3] Citing the research by Davis, Kalisch linked patient noncompliance with the inability to confront Aesculapian authority directly, leading patients to reclaim their autonomy after they have left the doctor's office.

In their article, The Use and Abuse of Aesculapian Authority in Veterinary Medicine, Rollins describes how veterinary medicine has evolved in such a way that the

Aesculapian authority is becoming increasingly more relevant.[4] They describe the transition of veterinary medicine from a focus primarily on agriculture to one that centers on companion animals that has brought about a significant shift in the veterinarian's role within society. Historically, animals were valued mainly for their economic contributions; however, the modern view of animals as family members has necessitated a profound transformation in veterinary practice. This shift mirrors the societal evolution in the perception of animals, from utilitarian assets to beings with intrinsic value, deserving of care and compassion akin to human family members.[4–8] Consequently, veterinarians are increasingly adopting a model of care that is reminiscent of pediatricians, whereby the approach to treatment is not solely based on economic considerations but is also deeply influenced by ethical, moral, and emotional factors.[4]

This evolution underscores the growing relevance of Aesculapian authority within veterinary medicine, a concept once exclusive to human health care. Veterinarians navigate the complexities of medicine, animal care and welfare, and human welfare. This authority, while providing the power to make significant positive impacts on animal health, also carries with it the responsibility to wield such power judiciously and with an awareness of the broader social implications. Thus, the necessity for adopting culturally responsive care in veterinary medicine has become increasingly pronounced. The traditional model of Aesculapian authority, which has shaped the patient-physician relationship in human medicine, provides a valuable framework for understanding the dynamics at play in veterinary care. However, as we apply these principles to veterinary medicine, we must also navigate the unique challenges that arise in a field whereby the patients cannot articulate their needs, and the responsibility to communicate and understand lies heavily on the veterinarian and the pet owner.

Veterinarians, therefore, must exercise their authority with a profound sense of responsibility, recognizing the trust placed in them by pet owners.[6,9,10] Culturally responsive care in this context means acknowledging and integrating the diverse values, beliefs, and expectations of pet owners into veterinary practice. It involves a collaborative approach that respects the cultural nuances of pet ownership and seeks to use both scientific knowledge and the lived experiences of pet owners.

Currently, there is only one exploration of the Aesculapian authority in veterinary medicine that was found in the literature.[4] While the article by Rollin provides an original exploration of Aesculapian authority in veterinary medicine, it nevertheless has a significant gap in addressing the complexities of veterinarian-pet owner relationships. Rollin articulates the potential for the abuse of Aesculapian authority, such as referencing euthanasia decisions, research trials, and the ethical dilemma between a veterinarian's duty and financial incentives.[4] However, this discourse, while valuable, falls short in addressing the deeper layers of medical racism and violence as well as epistemic violence—a critical oversight given the contemporary understanding of the veterinarian-pet owner dynamic.

Epistemology is the theory of knowledge and understanding, especially regarding its methods, validity, scope, and the distinction between justified belief and opinion. It is the philosophic basis of how we know what we know or think we know, thus it underlies what people think, what they believe, and how they apply new information.[11] As stated by Berenstain and colleagues, "Epistemologies have power. They have the power not only to transform worlds but to create them. And the worlds that they create can be better or worse. For many people, the worlds they create are predictably and reliably deadly."[12] Epistemic violence, the structural devaluation, and suppression of alternative systems of knowledge deemed inferior by a dominant knowledge system that is self-perceived as more accurate or valuable, remains unexplored in Rollin's analysis.[13,14] This omission is significant, especially when considering the historical and ongoing mistrust between disadvantaged communities and the medical establishment. Examples of such mistrust stem from grievous historical abuses, such as: using Black bodies for medical experimentation, the targeting of Native American, African American, and Puerto Rican women for involuntary, coercive, and compulsory sterilization under early 20th-century eugenics laws, and infectious disease risk in Black communities being used historically as justification for forced home removals, increased police surveillance and violence, and unsolicited medical interventions.[15] These abuses have fostered a profound mistrust of medical authorities. For an in-depth discussion on topics such as epistemic violence and methods for reshaping research to minimize harm to these communities, please see Chapter from Veterinary Clinics: Small Animal Practice (September 2024) issue- "Diversity, Equity, and Inclusion in Veterinary Medicine, Part I" titled as *The Value of Qualitative Research in Diversity, Equity, and Inclusion.* It is important to note, however, that this mistrust is not limited to the human medical establishment and it has been hypothesized that this skepticism translates to mistrust toward veterinarians.[16,17]

DEMOGRAPHICS OF PET OWNERSHIP: DEBUNKING STEREOTYPES AND AFFIRMING THE UNIVERSAL HUMAN-ANIMAL BOND ACROSS RACE, ETHNICITY, AND INCOME LEVELS

The profound and multifactorial benefits of the human-animal bond have been long established and the body of evidence only continues to grow, with most pet owners considering their pets as family members.[18–21] According to the 2017 to 2018 AVMA Pet Ownership and Demographic Sourcebook,[22] perceptions of pets as family members—measured across dogs, cats, birds, and horses—show little variation by race/ethnicity or household income. However, the 2022 AVMA Pet Ownership and Demographic Sourcebook[6] shifts its focus from demographic categories to defining "types" of pet owners. These are categorized as (1) low key and child free; (2) pampered pets; (3) casual caretakers; (4) occupied owners; and (5) enthusiastic families. Notably, the "pampered pets" category—characterized by owners who believe "My pets are my world, so I value high-quality service"—includes individuals both in the lowest income bracket (under $25k) and the highest (more than $200k), making it the only category encompassing such a diverse income range. This diversity within a single category further solidifies the idea that the strength of the human-animal bond transcends household income.

As described by Decker Sparks and colleagues, the scientific literature and cultural understanding within veterinary medicine often assert that race and ethnicity are primary factors influencing the decision to use veterinary services, including spay and neuter procedures, for companion animals.[17,23–30] Many of these studies suffer from biased sampling, opaque data analysis methods, and the use of non-validated survey tools targeted at specific populations. Furthermore, some of the research has examined race and ethnicity only alongside a narrow range of other variables, such as perceptions of pets' roles in the household and in limited geographic areas, often assuming cultural uniformity across racial, ethnic, geographic, and socioeconomic groups.[17,23–27,29–35]

Recent studies challenge these earlier findings by showing that race and ethnicity are not primary determinants in using veterinary services.[17] Instead, barriers such as cost, accessibility, lack of education, and mistrust in veterinarian-client interactions play a more significant role.[16,17,36–39] Specifically, discussions around veterinarian-client communication often focus on issues of cost, ethics, and perceived judgments about the client's ability to provide care.

These findings underscore the need to revisit and critically assess long-standing beliefs about the cultural willingness of people of color to seek veterinary care and acknowledge that structural barriers are the predominant factors limiting access to veterinary services. It is imperative for care providers to understand that holding onto these unfounded assumptions not only perpetuates these barriers but also worsens outcomes for pets and their families. Additionally, these assumptions contribute to the enduring distrust among people of color toward the medical community, fueled by a history of systemic racism, inequality, stigma, and oppression in medicine and scientific research.[15] Although veterinary institutions do not share this specific history of ethical breaches, veterinary medicine is still widely regarded as part of the broader medical field. Consequently, as outlined by Decker Sparks and colleagues, the reluctance of marginalized communities of color to engage with veterinary services mirrors their documented and justified distrust of medical, public health, and social service providers.[17,40–42] By clinging to these unfounded assumptions, we only deepen the divide and hinder progress toward equitable veterinary care.[17]

By not acknowledging the historical context of medical abuse and the consequent skepticism among minority communities, there is a missed opportunity to understand and bridge the deep divides that impact the veterinarian-pet owner relationship. Addressing this gap requires a concerted effort to validate and integrate diverse forms of knowledge and healing practices within veterinary care, fostering an environment whereby all pet owners feel seen, heard, and respected.

VETERINARIANS AS TRUSTED CAREGIVERS

Despite the documented history of distrust in the broader medical community among marginalized groups, the veterinary profession continues to hold a high level of trust among the general public. According to Gallup's 2023 Honesty and Ethics poll, amidst a general decline in trust across 23 surveyed professions, veterinarians continue to command a remarkable level of public confidence.[9] This distinction underscores the unique position veterinarians hold in society.

The exploration of care dynamics within veterinary medicine has been further illuminated by the insightful research of James, who through 29 qualitative interviews, delved into clients' expectations of highly skilled professional care.[10] Their study, which spanned the experiences of clients interacting with clinical social workers and small animal veterinarians, revealed a compelling parallel between these seemingly disparate professions. Contrary to previous research that positioned social workers as providers of more intensive care labor to humans[43,44] and veterinarians as offering less intensive care labor to humans,[45,46] their findings highlight a significant commonality in the client-caregiver relationship across both fields.

Veterinarians, often perceived primarily as medical professionals devoid of the emotional labor inherent in human care professions, are increasingly recognized for the depth of empathy and understanding they bring to their practice. This shift is particularly evident in the field of small animal practice, whereby pets are frequently regarded as family members, and the emotional stakes are correspondingly high.[5–8,47]

The demographic evolution within the veterinary profession, notably the transition from a male-dominated field to one whereby women now constitute the majority, has also played a crucial role in reshaping perceptions of care in veterinary medicine.[45,48] Research indicates that this gender shift is positively received by clients, who associate female veterinarians with a natural propensity for compassion toward their pets.[45] Empirical studies, such as those by Shaw and colleagues[49] corroborate this perception, noting that female veterinarians tend to invest more time in communicating with clients and building rapport, further enhancing the trust and connection integral to effective veterinary care.

This emerging understanding of veterinary medicine, as highlighted by James' research, emphasizes the profession's dual commitment to both expert knowledge and emotional connection. Veterinarians navigate the delicate balance between addressing medical conditions with scientific knowledge while acknowledging the profound emotional bond between pets and their owners. In doing so, they affirm their status not only as trusted health care providers but also as empathetic caregivers who play a crucial role in supporting the well-being of both animals and their human families.

Their research provides illuminating insights into what clients expect from their care providers, particularly highlighting the nuanced expectations placed on veterinarians and clinical social workers. The study underscores a universal desire among clients for professionals who not only possess expert knowledge and technical skills but who also exhibit a capacity for empathy and emotional intimacy that feels natural and genuine.

Clients interviewed by James regarded both clinical social workers and small animal veterinarians as both care occupations and skilled professions. James found that clients harbored a deep-seated fear of a clinical approach devoid of warmth and empathy. The fear was that care workers might prioritize clinical distance over heartfelt care, especially in situations involving intimate issues or the care of beloved pets. Highlighting this notion, pet owners expressed a desire for veterinarians to invest time in understanding and appreciating their pets' unique personalities, fostering a sense of familiarity and personal rapport.

Interestingly, 11 of the 29 clients stated that they intentionally sought out professional care workers with whom they felt they shared some aspect of identity, such as gender, sexual orientation, or ethnicity, believing that this shared identity fostered mutual respect and eased communication.

In this pivotal research, James' study reveals that veterinarians are increasingly seen as care workers similar to social workers, in which veterinarians address clients' emotional, mental, and/or social welfare problems along with their pet's medical problems. This highlights the need for more qualitative research into understanding the dynamics between veterinarians and pet owners and pushing for the field to adopt ways to implement culturally responsive care.

THE ESSENTIAL ROLE OF CULTURALLY RESPONSIVE CARE IN VETERINARY MEDICINE

The importance of culturally responsive care as well as the implementation in veterinary medicine is largely underexplored. Despite the recognition of the importance of human health care and the increasing calls within veterinary medicine to improve on its lack of diversity, equity, and inclusion within the field, veterinary medicine faces a notable gap in research and literature on culturally responsive care. Consequently, we find ourselves in a position whereby extrapolation from human medicine, particularly from nursing, becomes necessary.

The calls for culturally responsive care within human health care, known under various names such as culturally competent care, intercultural competence, cultural opening, patient-centered care, and transcultural care, has been echoed across numerous reports and standards in human health education and policy. The Institute of Medicine (IOM) underscored the significance of patient-centered care in its 2003 report on Health Professions Education, highlighting it as the foremost core competency for health professionals' education.[50,51] The U.S. Office of Minority Health has set national standards for culturally and linguistically appropriate health care services, stating that health care must "provide effective, equitable, understandable and respectful quality care and services that are responsive to diverse cultural health beliefs and practices, preferred languages, health literacy, and other communication needs."[52,53] Furthermore, the introduction of the National Culturally and Linguistically Appropriate Service Standards (CLAS Standards) in the United States in 2000, along with the Australian government's publication of "Cultural competency in health: A guide for policy, partnerships, and participation" in 2005, has marked significant strides toward embedding cultural competency in health care provision and policy.[54,55]

International calls for cultural openness in health care, such as the German federal government's demand for the "cultural opening" of health care facilities in 2007 and the NHS's migrant health guide offered since 2014, reflect a global acknowledgment of the necessity for culturally competent care.[54,56] These initiatives highlight how the field of human health care is centering culturally responsive care as a topic of vital importance. As veterinarians are seen more and more as professional care workers by society, the more critical it becomes within the field.

CULTURALLY RESPONSIVE CARE DEFINED

Before diving into the components of culturally responsive care, we must first understand and define racism, diversity, and culture as well as the concepts of cultural competency and cultural humility. It is also important to note that there is no universally used term for culturally responsive care, and while each term reflects varying nuances, they are linked by common core principles. In the subsequent section, the most commonly used terms will be defined. Later this article will detail the components of culturally responsive care that recur frequently in the literature, thereby providing a comprehensive understanding of the core components.

The American Nurses Association defines racism as "assaults on the human spirit in the form of biases, prejudices and an ideology of superiority that persistently cause moral suffering and perpetuate injustices and inequities."[57,58] The standard definition of culture in anthropology is "that complex whole which includes knowledge, belief, arts, morals, law, custom, and many other capabilities and habits acquired by man as a member of society."[59] Thus, as Schim and colleagues put it, "Culture is an individual concept, a group phenomenon, and an organizational reality."[60]

The concepts of cultural humility and cultural competence are overlapping yet distinct from one another. In the context of health care, cultural humility encompasses entering into a relationship with another person with the intention of honoring their beliefs, customs, and values. It acknowledges that this work is a lifelong ongoing process that requires constant self-reflection, identifying one's implicit biases, and the humility to learn from others. Cultural humility emphasizes addressing power imbalances, promotion of interpersonal sensitivity and openness, and an appreciation of intracultural variation and individuality to avoid stereotyping, all of which are known to promote patient-centered care.[52,61–63] On the other hand, cultural competence is conceptualized as a skill that can be taught, trained, and achieved and is often described as sufficient for working with diverse patients. The presumption is that if one has knowledge about another culture, the greater culturally competent care can be provided.[52] For example, culturally competent health workers feature components such as cultural awareness, knowledge, and skill. However, to quote Stubbe and colleagues, "Health care professionals need both process (cultural humility) and product (cultural competence) to interact effectively with culturally diverse patients.[52,64] Culturally competent care and culturally congruent care appear to be the most frequently used terms in the literature.

Please refer to the following summary of terms commonly associated with the concept of culturally responsive care.

- *Culturally congruent care:* Leininger, who created Leininger's Theory of Nursing: Cultural Care Diversity and Universality defines this as helping, supporting, facilitating, or empowering cognition-based actions or decisions, which are congruent with the cultural values, beliefs, and lifestyle of individuals, groups, or organizations.[65,66]
- *Culturally competent care:* This term has been defined in many ways. Alligood defined it as the creative, sensitive, and meaningful culture-based use of health and care knowledge to coordinate the needs and the usual ways of living of individuals or groups for acquiring meaningful health and well-being or coping with illnesses, disorders, and death.[67] Sharifi and colleagues define culturally competent nurses as ones who have the necessary sensitivity, knowledge, skill, and proficiency to act with cultural awareness. They have expert knowledge of different cultural practices, cultural humility, cultural assessments, and communication.[65]
- *Diversity-competent health professionals:* Defined as professionals that respect patients' unique attributes, are self-aware of biases, strive for equitable treatment using a human rights-based approach, and have a deep understanding of social determinants of health. They communicate effectively, listen empathetically, address individual needs collaboratively, and professionally collaborate with interpreters. This minimal definition contains basic elements such as respect, empathy, awareness, self-reflection, and communication skills that are known from other diversity and cultural competence definitions in health care.[68]
- *Cross-cultural competence*: This is defined as the ability to effectively perform in another culture. This ability requires the comparison or the encounter of two or more cultures. Cross-cultural competence facilitates the development of cultural competence.[65,69]
- *Patient-centered care:* This is defined as respecting and responding to individual patient's care needs, preferences, and values in all clinical decisions.[65,70]
- *Patient-centered communication:* This is defined as a process that invites and encourages patients and their families to actively participate and negotiate in decision-making about their care needs.[50,71]

Having established the common terms and definitions associated with culturally responsive care, it is crucial to understand what happens in its absence. The failure to implement culturally responsive practices can have far-reaching consequences, affecting both patient outcomes and the overall efficacy of the health care system.

CORE COMPONENTS OF CULTURALLY RESPONSIVE CARE

As the field of veterinary medicine increasingly acknowledges the significance of increased diversity, equity, and inclusion within the field and thus culturally responsive care, it becomes vital that we look to the literature on human health care. This section aims to synthesize the literature on culturally competent care, culturally congruent care, diversity competent care, and patient-centered care, providing a comprehensive overview of the essential elements that underpin these practices. It is to be noted, however, that while key components such as cultural awareness, knowledge, and skill are foundational; research consistently highlights that the true efficacy of these interactions often hinges on the health care provider's level of cultural humility.[68]

Furthermore, it is crucial to recognize that the responsibility for providing culturally responsive care does not rest solely on individual health care workers. Organizational involvement plays a critical role, as health care settings must actively support and implement policies that make the entire system culturally responsive.

Sharifi and colleagues's concept analysis of cultural competence in nursing provided critical insights into its defining attributes of cultural competence and necessary antecedents. The study identified the most common defining attributes of cultural competence as cultural awareness, cultural knowledge, cultural sensitivity, cultural skill, cultural proficiency, and dynamicity. See these concepts summarized later in discussion.[65]

- *Cultural Awareness:* Awareness is a cognitive construct, it requires not only knowing a fact or set of facts but knowledge and recognition (rethinking) of those facts.[60] In the review by Vaismoradi and colleagues it was discovered that education had an influence on the development of racism toward patients through hidden curricula and by learning in the workplace.[72] Thus, cultural awareness often happens during informal nursing education as direct education may not provide sufficient opportunities for nurses to become culturally aware.[72–74] Cultural awareness includes knowledge about the pervasive effects of culture on everyday life, experiences, and the interpretation of events. Knowledge about professional and organizational cultures is extremely useful, as is knowledge about one's own cultural heritage and present context.[60] It is not uncommon for people to be unaware that their beliefs or attitudes are not universal, and this unfounded assumption of universality leads to bias and assumptions of the motivations of those from other cultures. Thus, cultural awareness helps individuals assess their biases and prejudices and forms a basis for valuing others' beliefs and values.[65,75,76] In the absence of cultural awareness, one may impose the beliefs, values, and behavioral patterns of their own culture on people from other cultures.[77]
- *Cultural Knowledge*: Continuous information acquisition about different cultures as the basis for cultural understanding.[65,78] This entails integrating their medical knowledge about health-related beliefs, cultural values, incidence and prevalence of illnesses, and treatment effectiveness. This knowledge helps health care providers understand how patients think and behave during illness, and which matters should be noticed while making group caring decisions for patients from different ethnic groups.[65,77]
- *Cultural Sensitivity:* This is an affective or attitudinal construct related to a person's attitude about themselves and others, as well as their openness to learning along cultural dimensions.[60] Cultural sensitivity guides one to approach a patient or a community with humility by taking a learner's role rather than assuming a position of sufficient knowledge regarding any particular group.[60,79] This includes the understanding of the individual's personal cultural heritage, the disciplinary heritage into which one has been socialized as a health care provider, and the organizational culture in which one works.[60] This includes knowledge, attention, understanding, respect, and optimization of interventions based on patients' cultural needs.[65,80,81] It is utilized to help nurses understand how patients' attitudes and viewpoints affect their behaviors and care-seeking patterns.[65,82]
- *Cultural Skill:* The ability to establish effective communication with individuals from other cultures. Thus, one's ability to collect the relevant cultural knowledge

and then translate that information into effective client/patient interactions. This involves skills when it comes to communication, medical tasks, and decision-making.[83]

- *Cultural Proficiency:* Purposefully seeking out new cultural knowledge and skills and sharing them through articles, educational programs, and other methods; reflecting a commitment to change.[65,84]
- *Dynamicity:* A [health care provider] becomes culturally competent through frequent encounters with diverse patients.[65,85,86] This concept acknowledges that this is a dynamic process, not a set point, as people, cultures, and situations are always changing. An understanding of this dynamicity gives health care professionals an important perspective.

Interestingly, Sharifi and colleagues's concept analysis also found that there were necessary antecedents of cultural competence including cultural diversity, cultural encounter and interaction, cultural desire, cultural humility, general humanistic competencies, educational preparation, and organizational support. See these concepts summarized later in discussion.

- *Cultural Diversity:* Cultural diversity is a construct that varies in quantity and quality across place and time, including within health care organizations. Thus, accurate and current assessments of the state of cultural diversity within a health care organization is essential to ensure that suitable protocols are developed.[60] Additionally, it has been shown that diversities in nurses' cultural backgrounds is advantageous for the health care system in terms of improving the quality of patient care and the health care economy.[72,87]
- *Cultural Encounter and Interaction:* Interpersonal contacts and relationships among people from different cultures. Multiple studies have found that nurses cannot acquire cultural competence through self-study or other academic work; rather, they need to develop their personal and professional interactions with patients of different cultures. It is found that only through these direct interactions can they correct their own beliefs about different cultures and avoid prejudicial behaviors.[65,88–90]
- *Cultural Desire:* This refers to an internal desire within one's self to be culturally competent, it indicates that there is an enthusiasm for being open and flexible to others, accepting differences, and learning from others.[65,91]
- *Cultural Humility:* Cultural humility is a term attributed to Tervalon and Murray-Garcia who defined it as a process of "committing to an ongoing relationship with patients, communities, and colleagues" that requires "humility as individuals continually engage in self-reflection and self-critique."[61] As expanded by Fisher-Borne et al., "Cultural humility takes into account the fluidity and subjectivity of culture and challenges both individuals and institutions to address inequalities…emphasizing the need for accountability, not only on an individual level but also on an institutional level."[92] It is found that cultural humility fosters mutual empowerment, respect, collaboration, ideal care, and lifelong learning about patients from different cultures.[65,93,94]
- *General Humanistic Competencies:* In the field of nursing, there have been general competencies identified as necessary for nursing practice in all cultures and contexts. These are identified as positive personality characteristics, humanistic attitude, empathy, kindness, and respect.[65,95,96]
- *Educational Preparation:* It has been documented that participating in workshops and courses can develop nurses' cultural knowledge, insight, and skill and that

nurses with limited educational preparation avoid patients from different cultures.[65,97–99]

- *Organizational Support:* It has been established that the delivery of culturally congruent care and the fulfillment of the needs of ethnic minorities cause challenges that cannot be managed without the support of health care organizations.[65,100] Additionally, there have been multiple calls within the literature for health care organizations need to modify their philosophy, mission, goal, and vision and provide nurses with the necessary tools, recourses, and motives to care for patients from different cultures.[65,101,102]

Building on the foundational insights provided by Sharifi and colleagues, Schim and colleagues, and Vaismoradi and colleagues, we shift our focus to the work of Handtke and colleagues, who adopted a bottom-up approach in their research. Their methodology was aimed at extracting the components and strategies of culturally competent care directly from health care interventions designed specifically for culturally and linguistically diverse patients (CLDPs). Their scoping review was structured to not only gather these components and strategies from evaluated interventions but also to assess their impact on selected outcome measures. The goal of their study was to organize the identified elements into a coherent model of culturally competent health care provision.[54]

Their review pulled components and strategies of 67 culturally competent health care interventions, and clustered them into 20 subcategories of components, which were then grouped into 4 categories: (1) Components of culturally competent health care within facilities–Individual level; (2) Components of culturally competent health care within facilities–Organizational level; (3) Specific strategies to provide access to culturally competent health care; (4) Strategies to implement culturally competent health care within facilities. The following overview, adopted from their work, will summarize the components within each of these 4 major groups, providing a broad picture of how culturally competent care can be structured and implemented (**Table 1**). They illustrate the significant benefits these interventions have on health care outcomes. For veterinary professionals and organizations looking to integrate similar culturally competent strategies, a detailed examination of Handtke and colleagues's findings is recommended. Exploring this article can offer valuable insights and inspire thoughtful adaptation of these practices within the field of veterinary medicine.

Table 1
Components and strategies for culturally competent healthcare

Individual-Level Components	Linguistic/Cultural Matching of Providers, Culturally Specific Integration, Cultural and Linguistic Appropriate Materials, Involving Family
Organizational-Level Components	Cultural Competence Training, HR Development, Interpreter Services, Environmental Adaptation, Data Collection and Management
Implementation Strategies	Needs Assessment and Monitoring, Position/Group Creation, Action Planning, Leadership Involvement and Support, Promoting Structural Changes within the Organization
Access Strategies	Integration of Community Health Workers, Telemedicine, Using Different Outreach Methods, Developing Community Health Networks

Data from Handtke O, Schilgen B, Mösko M. Culturally competent health care – A scoping review of strategies implemented in healthcare organizations and a model of culturally competent health care provision. PLOS ONE. 2019;14(7):e0219971. https://doi.org/10.1371/journal.pone.0219971.

This study concludes with the logical argument that the most valuable way forward is to view culturally competent care as a complex intervention as this perspective can (1) enable due attention to the interacting micro-meso-macro levels of influences on individual and organizational practices and (2) inform the development of implementation strategies at each level.[54]

Similarly, Kwame and colleagues's review on patient-centered care and communication in nurse-patient interactions names facilitators and barriers that reflect the reviews noted above. Facilitators include: overcoming practical communication barriers in the nurse-patient dyad (such as using translators), acknowledging that while promptly managing medical tasks is crucial–the power of active listening is meaningful and therapeutic,[71,103] understanding patients and their unique needs,[104] showing empathy and attending attitudes,[71,103] expressing warmth and respect,[105] sharing information and inviting their opinion, and health policy that is oriented toward health care practices that facilitate patient-centered care and communication. Barriers identified in Kwame and colleagues's review include: Shortage of nursing staff, high workload, burnout, institutional level emphasis on task-centered care instead of on satisfying a patients' needs and preferences (this is acknowledged in several studies),[71,105–108] management styles as managers can either facilitate or impede patient-centered care,[105,108] and the environment of the care setting.[50,109] This review emphasized skills that cannot necessarily be taught are vital, such as empathy and attending attitudes as well as expressing warmth and respect. This review also adds to the literature the essential component of institutional-level involvement in successful patient-centered care, such as institutional emphasis on care centered on satisfying a patient's needs and preferences along with the management styles of the institution.

To conclude the summary of the research, we will end this section with Ziegler and colleagues', "Diversity Competence in Healthcare: Experts' Views on the Most Important Skills in Caring for Migrant and Minority Patients." This study included the expert opinion of 31 clinical and academic migrant health experts from 13 European countries who were asked the question, "What knowledge, attitudes and skills are most important to enable health professionals to take equally good care of all patients in evermore diverse, modern societies that include migrant and (ethnic) minority patients?" The results in this article found a higher level of disagreement between experts on knowledge content than on the importance of effective and especially pragmatic objectives. In fact, no solely knowledge-based competence made the high-priority ranking list. The authors theorize that this may imply that "knowledge" is considered less important overall than attitudes, reflection skills, and to a certain extent, practical skills.[68]

IMPLICATIONS OF INADEQUATE CULTURALLY RESPONSIVE CARE

The documented ramifications of inadequate culturally responsive care within human medicine are far-reaching and devastating. In Vaismoradi and colleagues' scoping review of racism in the nurse-patient relationship, they summarize that, "racism is the main cause of the patient's harm."[72] They summarize the findings of numerous studies that depict the multifaceted levels of harm caused by racism in health care. Stanley and colleagues found that patients who experienced racist discriminations often have poor health care outcomes and access to health care, and additionally suffer from mental health issues.[110] Hall and colleagues and Sim and colleagues both found in their research that racism in the form of implicit racial bias can be pervasively observed in the relationship between patients and health care providers, leading to health care disparities.[111,112] Powell and colleagues, Pugh and colleagues, and Rhee and colleagues found that racism within health care can hinder appropriate and adequate use of health care, following up with screening programs and preventative behaviors, adherence to the therapeutic regimen, and trust in the health care providers.[113–115] Moreover, Rogers and colleagues found that racism leads to the development of new disabilities in patients or can worsen the current disability of the patient.[116] Alarmingly, it was found in Vaismoradi and colleagues' review that racism with a nurse caused patients to distrust the whole health care system and eroded the relationship between that patient and nonracist nurses.[117] The consequence of this subset of patients developing a negative perspective of the whole health care system is is found that those patients go on to display disappointment and/or anger toward all nurses, which damages the sense of justice and pride among those nurses who did their best to provide equitable care to patients.[118] This implies a vicious feedback loop of hurt, distrust, and anger between health care professionals and their patients.

Ultimately, the research finds that persons in racial and ethnic minority groups were found to receive lower-quality health care than whites received, even when they were insured to the same degree and when other health care access-related factors, such as the ability to pay for care, were the same.[52,119] It is also found in the research that those patients in minority groups were also not getting their needs met in mental health treatment.[52,120,121]

After exploring the implications of inadequate culturally responsive care, it is equally important to illuminate the positive impacts of implementing such practices effectively. This shift in focus from the negative consequences to the affirmative benefits allows us to fully appreciate the transformative potential of culturally responsive care within veterinary medicine. Now, let us examine how embracing culturally responsive care can enhance patient outcomes, foster greater client satisfaction, and contribute to a more inclusive and effective health care environment.

ADVANTAGES OF IMPLEMENTING CULTURALLY RESPONSIVE CARE IN VETERINARY MEDICINE

The benefits of implementing culturally responsive care in human medicine are both vast and impactful, suggesting the impact it could make in veterinary medicine. As we transition from understanding the potential pitfalls of neglecting such care, it becomes increasingly clear that the advantages extend far beyond the immediate health outcomes of patients. In this section, we will explore the multifaceted benefits of culturally responsive care, underscoring why it is vital to incorporate it into modern veterinary practice.

There is a tremendous amount of research within human health care underlining the multifaceted and expansive benefits of culturally responsive care. Starting with the benefits of effective communication, studies have shown that respectful communication between nurses and patients can reduce uncertainty, enhance greater patient engagement in decision-making, improve patient adherence to medication and treatment plans, and increase social support, safety, and patient satisfaction in care.[50,103,122] Sharifi and colleagues provide an extensive review of the documented benefits of culturally competent care including reduction in health care inequalities, patients developing greater trust in health care systems, greater adherence to treatment regimens, greater patient satisfaction, reduces health care costs, lowered morbidity and mortality rates, and consequently creates a better quality of life for patients.[65,69,79,123–128] Sharifi and colleagues additionally found in their review that culturally competent care creates a sense of cultural safety in their patients, referring to the recognition of the sociopolitical conditions of specific groups during care delivery in order to preserve their identities, consider their needs in care plans, impartially provide care services to them, and prevent them from feeling alienated and deprived of health care services.[65,129,130] It has been found in the literature that patients that experience the feeling of cultural safety can lead to strengthening their relationships with health care providers, improve their health-seeking behaviors, and enhancing their satisfaction with health care services.[65]

The benefits are not limited to patients but benefit the health care provider as well. Research shows that it facilitates nurses' mutual relationships and successful interactions with patients, gives nurses a feeling of respect and self-empowerment, and develops their personal and professional values, relationships, and performance.[65,78,124,127,128]

After thoroughly exploring the varied benefits of culturally responsive care in human health care, it is evident that the integration of these practices has the potential not only to improve health outcomes for animals but can also significantly enhance the satisfaction and trust of pet owners. These benefits are documented in human health care, whereby effective communication and culturally responsive care have been shown to reduce health care disparities, increase patient adherence, build trust, and create a better quality of life. Such outcomes underscore the need for a veterinary environment that is not only skilled in medical treatment but also proficient in culturally responsive practices.

As we advance this discussion, it is crucial to recognize that while there is no universally accepted term for culturally responsive care, the core principles remain consistent across various terminologies and frameworks. Each term, whether it refers to cultural competence, cultural humility, or patient-centered care, emphasizes the importance of understanding and respecting the diverse backgrounds of clients.

SUMMARY

As we conclude this article on culturally responsive care, it is imperative to reiterate that while the components outlined above are crucial in the journey toward embracing and implementing such care, they alone are not sufficient. Knowledge and skills, while foundational, must be complemented by deeper, more personal transformations in attitude and approach.

Institutional buy-in forms a critical backbone for the successful integration of culturally competent practices.[54,65,92,100–102,131,132] Organizations must not only endorse but actively promote and facilitate an environment whereby cultural sensitivity is woven into the very fabric of health care delivery. However, beyond the structural changes at the institutional level, the core of culturally responsive care lies in the individual practitioner's commitment to cultural humility.[52,68,92]

Moreover, it is essential to integrate culturally based education within veterinary school curriculums, particularly given the evidence from human nursing that education influences the development of racism toward patients through hidden curricula and workplace learning.[65,72,97,98,133]

Finally, increasing diversity within the field has been proven to improve the quality of care.[10,54,68,72,87] Professional care recipients often intentionally seek out health care workers with whom they feel a shared aspect of identity.[10] This highlights the importance of such diversity in building trust and enhancing service delivery.

Thus, to truly excel in providing culturally responsive care, veterinary professionals must integrate both the external components of knowledge and skills and the internal process of developing cultural humility.

DECLARATION OF ARTIFICIAL INTELLIGENCE AND ARTIFICIAL INTELLIGENCE-ASSISTED TECHNOLOGIES IN THE WRITING PROCESS

During the preparation of this study, the author used ChatGPT4 in order to improve readability. After using this tool, the author reviewed and edited the content as needed and takes full responsibility for the content of the publication.

REFERENCES

1. Kalisch BJ. Of half gods and mortals: Aesculapian authority. Nurs Outlook 1975; 23(1):22–8.
2. Siegler M, Osmond H. Models of madness, models of medicine. The University of Michigan; Macmillan; 1974.
3. Davis MS. Variations in patients' compliance with doctors' advice: an empirical analysis of patterns o communication. Am J Public Health Nation's Health 1968; 58(2):274. https://doi.org/10.2105/ajph.58.2.274.
4. Rollin BE. The use and abuse of Aesculapian authority in veterinary medicine. J Am Vet Med Assoc 2002;220(8):1144–9. https://doi.org/10.2460/javma.2002. 220.1144.
5. Brown A. About half of U.S. pet owners say their pets are as much a part of their family as a human member. Pew Research Center. Available at: https://www. pewresearch.org/short-reads/2023/07/07/about-half-us-of-pet-owners-say-their-pets-are-as-much-a-part-of-their-family-as-a-human-member/. Accessed April 8, 2024.
6. American Veterinary Medical Association. AVMA 2022 pet ownership and demographic Sourcebook. 2022. Available at: https://ebusiness.avma.org/Product Catalog/product.aspx?ID=2050. Accessed April 8, 2024.
7. Ryan S, Ziebland S. On interviewing people with pets: reflections from qualitative research on people with long-term conditions. Sociol Health Illness 2015; 37(1):67–80. https://doi.org/10.1111/1467-9566.12176.
8. Charles N, Davies CA. My family and other animals: pets as kin. Socio Res Online 2008;13(5):13–26. https://doi.org/10.5153/sro.1798.
9. Gallup. Honesty/ethics in professions. Gallup.com 2006. Available at: https://news.gallup.com/poll/1654/Honesty-Ethics-Professions.aspx. Accessed April 8, 2024.
10. James AFF. Expert knowledge or emotional connection? Examining clients' expectations for highly-skilled professional care. Socio Spectr 2021;41(5):407–21. https://doi.org/10.1080/02732173.2021.1945514.
11. Hoag J. Research guides @ fordham: information literacy : epistemology. Available at: https://fordham.libguides.com/InformationLiteracy/Epistemology. Accessed April 9, 2024.
12. Berenstain N, Dotson K, Paredes J, et al. Epistemic oppression, resistance, and resurgence. Contemp Polit Theory 2022;21(2):283–314. https://doi.org/10.1057/s41296-021-00483-z.
13. Pérez M. Epistemic violence: reflections between the invisible and the ignorable. El lugar sin límites 2019;1(1):81–98.
14. Elías S. Epistemic violence against indigenous peoples. Debates Indígenas. 2020. Available at: https://debatesindigenas.org/en/2020/08/01/epistemic-violence-against-indigenous-peoples/. Accessed April 9, 2024.
15. Nuriddin A, Mooney G, White AIR. Reckoning with histories of medical racism and violence in the USA. Lancet 2020;396(10256):949–51. https://doi.org/10.1016/S0140-6736(20)32032-8.

16. Park RM, Gruen ME, Royal K. Association between dog owner demographics and decision to seek veterinary care. Veterinary Sciences 2021;8(1):7. https://doi.org/10.3390/vetsci8010007.

17. Decker Sparks JL, Camacho B, Tedeschi P, et al. Race and ethnicity are not primary determinants in utilizing veterinary services in underserved communities in the United States. J Appl Anim Welfare Sci 2018;21(2):120–9. https://doi.org/10.1080/10888705.2017.1378578.

18. Jenkins JL, Rudd ML. Decolonizing animal welfare through a social justice framework. Front Vet Sci 2022;8. Available at: https://www.frontiersin.org/articles/10.3389/fvets.2021.787555. Accessed August 17, 2022.

19. Companions and animals for reform and equity, harvard project implicit. Companions and animals for reform and equity. 2020. Available at: https://careawo.org/wp-content/uploads/2021/07/ProjectImplicited.pdf.

20. Hawes SM, Hupe T, Morris KN. Punishment to support: the need to align animal control enforcement with the human social justice movement. Animals 2020;10(10):1902. https://doi.org/10.3390/ani10101902.

21. Arkow P. Human–animal relationships and social work: opportunities beyond the veterinary environment. Child Adolesc Soc Work J 2020;37(6):573–88. https://doi.org/10.1007/s10560-020-00697-x.

22. American Veterinary Medical Association. 2017-2018 AVMA Pet Ownership and Demographic Sourcebook. Schaumburg (IL): American Veterinary Medial Association; 2019.

23. Baumann MR. San antonio animal care services project 2007: summary findings & related policy implications. Available at: https://webapps1.sanantonio.gov/rfcadocs/R_2064_20070810092030.pdf.

24. Faver CA. Sterilization of companion animals: exploring the attitudes and behaviors of latino students in south Texas. J Appl Anim Welfare Sci 2009;12(4):314–30. https://doi.org/10.1080/10888700903163534.

25. Hosey G, Melfi V. Human-animal interactions, relationships and bonds: a review and analysis of the literature. Int J Comp Psychol 2014;27(1). https://doi.org/10.46867/ijcp.2014.27.01.01.

26. Ortega-Pacheco A, Rodriguez-Buenfil JC, Bolio-Gonzalez ME, et al. A survey of dog populations in urban and rural areas of yucatan, Mexico. Anthrozoös 2007;20(3):261–74. https://doi.org/10.2752/089279307X224809.

27. Risley-Curtiss C, Holley LC, Wolf S. The animal-human bond and ethnic diversity. Soc Work 2006;51(3):257–68. https://doi.org/10.1093/sw/51.3.257.

28. Schoenfeld-Tacher RM, Kogan LR. Professional veterinary programs' perceptions and experiences pertaining to emotional support animals and service animals, and recommendations for policy development. J Vet Med Educ 2017;44(1):166–78. https://doi.org/10.3138/jvme.0116-003R.

29. Trevejo R, Yang M, Lund EM. Epidemiology of surgical castration of dogs and cats in the United States. J Am Vet Med Assoc 2011. https://doi.org/10.2460/javma.238.7.898.

30. Wolf CA, Lloyd JW, Black JR. An examination of US consumer pet-related and veterinary service expenditures, 1980–2005. J Am Vet Med Assoc 2008. https://doi.org/10.2460/javma.233.3.404.

31. Chu K, Anderson WM, Rieser MY. Population characteristics and neuter status of cats living in households in the United States. J Am Vet Med Assoc 2009. https://doi.org/10.2460/javma.234.8.1023.

32. Landau RE, Beck A, Glickman LT, et al. Use of veterinary services by Latino dog and cat owners with various degrees of English-language proficiency. J Am Vet Med Assoc 2016. https://doi.org/10.2460/javma.248.6.681.

33. Schoenfeld-Tacher R, Kogan LR, Wright ML. Comparison of strength of the human-animal bond between Hispanic and non-Hispanic owners of pet dogs and cats. J Am Vet Med Assoc 2010. https://doi.org/10.2460/javma.236.5.529.

34. Poss JE, Bader JO. Attitudes toward companion animals among hispanic residents of a Texas border community. J Appl Anim Welfare Sci 2007;10(3):243–53. https://doi.org/10.1080/10888700701353717.

35. Poss JE, Bader JO. Results of a free spay/neuter program in a hispanic colonia on the Texas-Mexico border. J Appl Anim Welfare Sci 2008;11(4):346–51. https://doi.org/10.1080/10888700802330010.

36. LaVallee E, Mueller MK, McCobb E. A systematic review of the literature addressing veterinary care for underserved communities. J Appl Anim Welfare Sci 2017; 20(4):381–94 https://doi.org/10.1080/10888705.2017.1337515.

37. Humane Society of the United States. Pets for life: a new community understanding. 2012. Available at: https://www.humanesociety.org/sites/default/files/docs/2012-pets-for-life-report.pdf. Accessed February 26, 2020.

38. Poss J, Everett M. Impact of a bilingual mobile spay/neuter clinic in a U.S./Mexico border city. J Appl Anim Welfare Sci : JAAWS 2006;9:71–7. https://doi.org/10.1207/s15327604jaws0901_7.

39. King E, Mueller MK, Dowling-Guyer S, et al. Financial fragility and demographic factors predict pet owners' perceptions of access to veterinary care in the United States. J Am Vet Med Assoc 2022;260(14):1–8. https://doi.org/10.2460/javma.21.11.0486.

40. Armstrong K, Ravenell KL, McMurphy S, et al. Racial/ethnic differences in physician distrust in the United States. Am J Publ Health 2007;97(7):1283–9. https://doi.org/10.2105/AJPH.2005.080762.

41. Corbie-Smith G. The continuing legacy of the tuskegee syphilis study; considerations for clinical investigation. Am J Med Sci 1999;317(1):5–8. https://doi.org/10.1016/S0002-9629(15)40464-1.

42. Corbie-Smith G, Thomas SB, St. George DMM. Distrust, race, and research. Arch Intern Med 2002;162(21):2458–63. https://doi.org/10.1001/archinte.162.21.2458.

43. Occupational outlook handbook, 2016–17 edition, social workers. 2015. Available at: https://www.bls.gov/ooh/community-and-social-service/social-workers.htm. Accessed April 21, 2024.

44. National Association of Social Workers Center for Workforce Studies. Assuring the sufficiency of a frontline workforce: a national study of licensed social workers, executive summary. Available at: http://workforce.socialworkers.org/studies/nasw_06_execsummary.pdf. Accessed April 21, 2024.

45. Irvine L, Vermilya JR. Gender work in a feminized profession: the case of veterinary medicine. Gend Soc 2010;24(1):56–82. https://doi.org/10.1177/0891243209355978.

46. Podberscek AL, Paul ES, Serpell JA. Companion animals and us: exploring the relationships between people and pets. New York: Cambridge University Press; 2000. p. 335, xi.

47. Podberscek AL, Paul ES, Serpell JA. Companion Animals and Us: Exploring the Relationships between People and Pets. Cambridge University Press; 2000. p. 335, xi.

48. Lincoln AE. The shifting supply of men and women to occupations: feminization in veterinary education. Soc Forces 2010;88(5):1969–98.
49. Shaw JR, Bonnett BN, Roter DL, et al. Gender differences in veterinarian-client-patient communication in companion animal practice. J Am Vet Med Assoc 2012;241(1):81–8. https://doi.org/10.2460/javma.241.1.81.
50. Kwame A, Petrucka PM. A literature-based study of patient-centered care and communication in nurse-patient interactions: barriers, facilitators, and the way forward. BMC Nurs 2021;20(1):158. https://doi.org/10.1186/s12912-021-00684-2.
51. Long KA. The institute of medicine report health professions education: a bridge to quality. Pol Polit Nurs Pract 2003;4(4):259. https://doi.org/10.1177/1527154403258304.
52. Stubbe DE. Practicing cultural competence and cultural humility in the care of diverse patients. FOC 2020;18(1):49–51. https://doi.org/10.1176/appi.focus.20190041.
53. National Standards for Culturally and Linguistically Appropriate Services in Health Care. Final report. 2001. Available at: https://thinkculturalhealth.hhs.gov/assets/pdfs/EnhancedNationalCLASStandards.pdf.
54. Handtke O, Schilgen B, Mösko M. Culturally competent healthcare – a scoping review of strategies implemented in healthcare organizations and a model of culturally competent healthcare provision. PLoS One 2019;14(7):e0219971. https://doi.org/10.1371/journal.pone.0219971.
55. National Health and Medical Research Council (Australia). Cultural Competency in Health: A Guide for Policy, Partnerships and Participation. Commonwealth of Australia; 2005. http://www.nhmrc.gov.au/publications/_files/hp19.pdf.
56. National Health Service. Migrant health guide. 2014. Available at: https://www.gov.uk/topic/health-protection/migrant-health-guide. Accessed April 21, 2024.
57. American Nurses Association. National Commission to address racism in nursing: defining racism. 2021. Available at: https://www.nursingworld.org/~49f737/globalassets/practiceandpolicy/workforce/commission-to-address-racism/final-defining-racism-june-2021.pdf. Accessed April 21, 2024.
58. United Nations Educational. Scientific, and Cultural Organization. UNESCO universal declaration on cultural diversity. 2004. Available at: http://portal/unesco.org/culture. Accessed April 21, 2024.
59. Tylor EB. Primitive culture. New York: Torchbooks; 1871.
60. Schim SM, Doorenbos A, Benkert R, et al. Culturally congruent care: putting the puzzle together. J Transcult Nurs 2007;18(2):103–10. https://doi.org/10.1177/1043659606298613.
61. Tervalon M, Murray-García J. Cultural humility versus cultural competence: a critical distinction in defining physician training outcomes in multicultural education. J Health Care Poor Underserved 1998;9(2):117–25. https://doi.org/10.1353/hpu.2010.0233.
62. Hunt LM. Beyond cultural competence: applying humility to clinical settings. In: The social medicine reader, vol. II, 3rd edition. Duke University Press; 2019. Available at: https://doi.org/10.1515/9781478004363-020. Accessed April 21, 2024.
63. Hook JN, Watkins CE, Davis DE, et al. Cultural humility in psychotherapy supervision. APT 2016;70(2):149–66. https://doi.org/10.1176/appi.psychotherapy.2016.70.2.149.
64. Yancu C, Farmer DF. Product or process: cultural competence or cultural humility? Palliative Medicine and Hospice Care 2017;3(1). https://doi.org/10.17140/PMHCOJ-3-e005.

65. Sharifi N, Adib-Hajbaghery M, Najafi M. Cultural competence in nursing: a concept analysis. Int J Nurs Stud 2019;99:103386. https://doi.org/10.1016/j.ijnurstu.2019.103386.

66. Leininger MM. The theory of culture care and the ethnonursing research method. In: Transcultural nursing: concepts, Theories, research & practice. New York: McGraw-Hill; 2002. p. 71–116.

67. Alligood MR. Nursing theorists and their work. USA: Elsevior; 2014.

68. Ziegler S, Michaëlis C, Sørensen J. Diversity competence in healthcare: experts' views on the most important skills in caring for migrant and minority patients. Societies 2022;12(2):43. https://doi.org/10.3390/soc12020043.

69. Cai DY. A concept analysis of cultural competence. Int J Nurs Sci 2016;3(3): 268–73. https://doi.org/10.1016/j.ijnss.2016.08.002.

70. Institute of Medicine (US) Committee on Quality of Health Care in America. Crossing the quality chasm: a new health system for the 21st century. National Academies Press (US); 2001. Available at: http://www.ncbi.nlm.nih.gov/books/NBK222274/. Accessed April 21, 2024.

71. McCabe C. Nurse-patient communication: an exploration of patients' experiences. J Clin Nurs 2004;13(1):41–9. https://doi.org/10.1111/j.1365-2702.2004.00817.x.

72. Vaismoradi M, Fredriksen Moe C, Ursin G, et al. Looking through racism in the nurse–patient relationship from the lens of culturally congruent care: a scoping review. J Adv Nurs 2022;78(9):2665–77. https://doi.org/10.1111/jan.15267.

73. Hultsjö S, Bachrach-Lindström M, Safipour J, et al. "Cultural awareness requires more than theoretical education" - nursing students' experiences. Nurse Educ Pract 2019;39:73–9. https://doi.org/10.1016/j.nepr.2019.07.009.

74. Kaihlanen AM, Hietapakka L, Heponiemi T. Increasing cultural awareness: qualitative study of nurses' perceptions about cultural competence training. BMC Nurs 2019;18(1):38. https://doi.org/10.1186/s12912-019-0363-x.

75. Leonard BJ, Plotnikoff GA. Awareness: the heart of cultural competence. AACN Adv Crit Care 2000;11(1):51–9.

76. Zander PE. Cultural competence: analyzing the construct. J Theor Construct Test 2007;11(2):50. Available at: https://openurl.ebsco.com/contentitem/gcd:32034407?sid=ebsco:plink:crawler&id=ebsco:gcd:32034407. Accessed April 22, 2024.

77. Campinha-Bacote J. Cultural competemility: a paradigm shift in the cultural competence versus cultural humility debate – Part I. OJIN: Online J Issues Nurs. 24(1). doi:10.3912/OJIN.Vol24No01PPT20.

78. Kim-Godwin YS, Clarke PN, Barton L. A model for the delivery of culturally competent community care. J Adv Nurs 2001;35(6):918–25. https://doi.org/10.1046/j.1365-2648.2001.01929.x.

79. Betancourt JR, Green AR, Carrillo JE, et al. Cultural competence and health care disparities: key perspectives and trends. Health Aff 2005;24(2):499–505. https://doi.org/10.1377/hlthaff.24.2.499.

80. Jirwe M, Gerrish K, Keeney S, et al. Identifying the core components of cultural competence: findings from a Delphi study. J Clin Nurs 2009;18(18):2622–34. https://doi.org/10.1111/j.1365-2702.2008.02734.x.

81. Foronda CL. A concept analysis of cultural sensitivity. J Transcult Nurs 2008; 19(3):207–12. https://doi.org/10.1177/1043659608317093.

82. Burchum JLR. Cultural competence: an evolutionary perspective. Nurs Forum 2002;37(4):5–15. https://doi.org/10.1111/j.1744-6198.2002.tb01287.x.

83. Marja SL, Suvi A. Cultural competence learning of the health care students using simulation pedagogy: an integrative review. Nurse Educ Pract 2021;52:103044. https://doi.org/10.1016/j.nepr.2021.103044.

84. Cross TL, Others A. Towards a culturally competent system of care: a monograph on effective services for minority children who are severely emotionally disturbed. CASSP technical assistance center, georgetown university child development center, 3800 reservoir rd. 1989. Available at: https://eric.ed.gov/?id=ED330171. Accessed April 22, 2024.

85. Capell J, Veenstra G, Dean E. Cultural competence in healthcare: critical analysis of the construct, its assessment and implications - ProQuest. J Theor Construct Test 2007;11(1):30–7.

86. Dunn AM. Culture competence and the primary care provider. J Pediatr Health Care 2002;16(3):105–11.

87. Gomez LE, Bernet P. Diversity improves performance and outcomes. J Natl Med Assoc 2019;111(4):383–92. https://doi.org/10.1016/j.jnma.2019.01.006.

88. Kardong-Edgren S, Campinha-Bacote J. Cultural competency of graduating US Bachelor of Science nursing students. Contemp Nurse 2008;28(1–2):37–44. https://doi.org/10.5172/conu.673.28.1-2.37.

89. Campinha-Bacote J. The process of cultural competence in the delivery of healthcare services: a model of care. J Transcult Nurs 2002;13(3):181–4. https://doi.org/10.1177/10459602013003003, discussion 200-201.

90. Khezerloo S, Mokhtari J. Cultural competency in nursing education: a review article. J Med Ethics Hist Med 2016;8(6):11–21.

91. Henderson S, Horne M, Hills R, et al. Cultural competence in healthcare in the community: a concept analysis. Health Soc Care Community 2018;26(4):590–603. https://doi.org/10.1111/hsc.12556.

92. Fisher-Borne M, Cain JM, Martin SL. From mastery to accountability: cultural humility as an alternative to cultural competence. Soc Work Educ 2015;34(2):165–81. https://doi.org/10.1080/02615479.2014.977244.

93. Steefel L, Foronda C, Baptiste DL, et al. Cultural humility: a concept analysis. J Transcult Nurs 2016;22(3):210–7.

94. Foronda C, Baptiste DL, Reinholdt MM, et al. Cultural humility: a concept analysis. J Transcult Nurs 2016;27(3):210–7. https://doi.org/10.1177/1043659615592677.

95. Dreher M, Macnaughton N. Cultural competence in nursing: foundation or fallacy? Nurs Outlook 2002;50(5):181–6. https://doi.org/10.1067/mno.2002.125800.

96. Jirwe M, Gerrish K, Emami A. The theoretical framework of cultural competence. J Multicult Nurs Health 2006;12(3).

97. Wells MI. Beyond cultural competence: a model for individual and institutional cultural development. J Community Health Nurs 2000;17(4):189–99. https://doi.org/10.1207/S15327655JCHN1704_1.

98. Beach MC, Price EG, Gary TL, et al. Cultural competence: a systematic review of health care provider educational interventions. Med Care 2005;43(4):356–73. https://doi.org/10.1097/01.mlr.0000156861.58905.96.

99. Songwathana P, Sriratanaprapat J. Cultural competency in professional nursing: some considerations for Thai nurses. Catalyst 2015;11(1):27.

100. Taylor R. Addressing barriers to cultural competence. J Nurses Staff Dev 2005;21(4):135–42. https://doi.org/10.1097/00124645-200507000-00001, quiz 143-144.

101. Chrisman NJ. Extending cultural competence through systems change: academic, hospital, and community partnerships. J Transcult Nurs 2007;18(1 Suppl):68S–76S. https://doi.org/10.1177/1043659606295692, discussion 77S-85S.

102. Taylor RA, Alfred MV. Nurses' perceptions of the organizational supports needed for the delivery of culturally competent care. West J Nurs Res 2010; 32(5):591–609. https://doi.org/10.1177/0193945909354999.

103. Bello O. Effective communication in nursing practice: a literature review. BSc Nursing Thesis. Arcada 2017. Available at:.

104. Camara BS, Belaid L, Manet H, et al. What do we know about patient-provider interactions in sub-Saharan Africa? a scoping review. The Pan African Medical Journal 2020;37(88). https://doi.org/10.11604/pamj.2020.37.88.24009.

105. Yoo HJ, Lim OB, Shim JL. Critical care nurses' communication experiences with patients and families in an intensive care unit: a qualitative study. PLoS One 2020;15(7):e0235694. https://doi.org/10.1371/journal.pone.0235694.

106. Murira N, Lützen K, Lindmark G, et al. Communication patterns between health care providers and their clients at an antenatal clinic in Zimbabwe. Health Care Women Int 2003;24(2):83–92. https://doi.org/10.1080/07399330390170060.

107. Loghmani L, Borhani F, Abbaszadeh A. The facilitators and barriers to communication between nurses and family member in intensive care unit in kerman, Iran. J Caring Sci 2013;3(1):67–82. https://doi.org/10.5681/jcs.2014.008.

108. McLean A. The person in dementia: a study of nursing home care in the us. University of Toronto Press; 2006. Available at: https://muse.jhu.edu/pub/50/monograph/book/104096. Accessed April 22, 2024.

109. Mastors P. What do patients want, need, and have the right to expect? Nurs Adm Q 2018;42(3):192–8. https://doi.org/10.1097/NAQ.0000000000000297.

110. Stanley J, Harris R, Cormack D, et al. The impact of racism on the future health of adults: protocol for a prospective cohort study. BMC Publ Health 2019;19(1): 346. https://doi.org/10.1186/s12889-019-6664-x.

111. Sim W, Lim WH, Ng CH, et al. The perspectives of health professionals and patients on racism in healthcare: a qualitative systematic review. PLoS One 2021; 16(8):e0255936. https://doi.org/10.1371/journal.pone.0255936.

112. Hall WJ, Chapman MV, Lee KM, et al. Implicit racial/ethnic bias among health care professionals and its influence on health care outcomes: a systematic review. Am J Publ Health 2015;105(12):e60–76. https://doi.org/10.2105/AJPH. 2015.302903.

113. Powell DL. Social determinants of health: cultural competence is not enough. Creat Nurs 2016;22(1):5–10. https://doi.org/10.1891/1078-4535.22.1.5.

114. Pugh M, Perrin PB, Rybarczyk B, et al. Racism, mental health, healthcare provider trust, and medication adherence among Black patients in safety-net primary care. J Clin Psychol Med Settings 2021;28(1):181–90. https://doi.org/10.1007/s10880-020-09702-y.

115. Rhee TG, Marottoli RA, Van Ness PH, et al. Impact of perceived racism on healthcare access among older minority adults. Am J Prev Med 2019;56(4): 580–5. https://doi.org/10.1016/j.amepre.2018.10.010.

116. Rogers SE, Thrasher AD, Miao Y, et al. Discrimination in healthcare settings is associated with disability in older adults: health and retirement study, 2008–2012. J Gen Intern Med 2015;30(10):1413–20. https://doi.org/10.1007/s11606-015-3233-6.

117. Benkert R, Hollie B, Nordstrom CK, et al. Trust, mistrust, racial identity and patient satisfaction in urban African American primary care patients of nurse practitioners. J Nurs Scholarsh 2009;41(2):211–9. https://doi.org/10.1111/j.1547-5069.2009.01273.x.

118. Debesay J, Kartzow AH, Fougner M. Healthcare professionals' encounters with ethnic minority patients: the critical incident approach. Nurs Inq 2022;29(1): e12421. https://doi.org/10.1111/nin.12421.

119. Institute of Medicine (US. Committee on understanding and eliminating racial and ethnic disparities in health care. In: Smedley BD, Stith AY, Nelson AR, editors. Unequal treatment: confronting racial and ethnic disparities in health care. National Academies Press (US); 2003. Available at: http://www.ncbi.nlm. nih.gov/books/NBK220358/. Accessed March 20, 2020.

120. Holden K, McGregor B, Thandi P, et al. Toward culturally centered integrative care for addressing mental health disparities among ethnic minorities. Psychol Serv 2014;11(4):357–68. https://doi.org/10.1037/a0038122.

121. Gonzales J, Papadopoulos A. Mental health disparities. In: Mental health services: a public health perspective. 2nd Edition. Oxford University Press; 2004. p. 474, xviii.

122. Ruben BD. Communication theory and health communication practice: the more things change, the more they stay the same. Health Commun 2016;31(1):1–11. https://doi.org/10.1080/10410236.2014.923086.

123. French BM. Culturally Competent Care: the awareness of self and others. J Infusion Nurs 2003;26(4):252–5. https://doi.org/10.1097/00129804-200307000-00011.

124. Smith LS. Reaching for cultural competence. Nursing 2013;43(6):30. https://doi. org/10.1097/01.NURSE.0000429794.17073.87.

125. Alizadeh S, Chavan M. Cultural competence dimensions and outcomes: a systematic review of the literature. Health Soc Care Community 2016;24(6): e117–30. https://doi.org/10.1111/hsc.12293.

126. Dudas KI. Cultural competence: an evolutionary concept analysis. Nurs Educ Perspect 2012;33(5):317.

127. Smith LS. Concept analysis: cultural competence. J Cult Divers 1998;5(1):4–10.

128. Suh EE. The model of cultural competence through an evolutionary concept analysis. J Transcult Nurs 2004;15(2):93–102. https://doi.org/10.1177/1043659 603262488.

129. Blanchet Garneau A, Pepin J. Cultural competence: a constructivist definition. J Transcult Nurs 2015;26(1):9–15. https://doi.org/10.1177/1043659614541294.

130. Bozorgzad P, Negarandeh R, Raiesifar A, et al. Cultural safety: an evolutionary concept analysis. Holist Nurs Pract 2016;30(1):33–8. https://doi.org/10.1097/ HNP.0000000000000125.

131. Narayan MC, Mallinson RK. Transcultural nurse views on culture-sensitive/patient-centered assessment and care planning: a descriptive study. J Transcult Nurs 2022;33(2):150–60. https://doi.org/10.1177/10436596211046986.

132. Werner JM, DeSimone RL. Human resource development. 4th edition. 2006. Available at: http://sutlib2.sut.ac.th/sut_contents/H96679.pdf.

133. Heidari MR, Anooshe M, Azadarmaki T, et al. Exploration of context of the cultural care education in Iran. J Nurs Educ 2013;1–8.

Allies, Advocates, and Accomplices in Veterinary Medicine

Issa Robson, BSc Animal Physiology, BVM&S, MRCVS, MSc Ruminant Nutrition[a,b,c,*]

KEYWORDS

• Allyship • Diversity • Inclusion • Equity • Discrimination • Veterinary

KEY POINTS

- Allyship can be seen as the continuous practice and activities of a person who supports the rights of a minority or marginalized group without being a member of that group.
- Allyship can be used as a tool to foster inclusive workplaces, leading to safer patient outcomes.
- Foundational allyship skills include becoming an independent learner, learning to regulate the difficult emotions that arise discussing inequity and building self-confidence to stand up to discriminatory and inappropriate behaviors.

DEFINITIONS
Marginalized

Marginalized community refers to groups of people who face discrimination and exclusion (social, political, and economic)[1] can include people with disabilities, who are neurodivergent, who have mental health conditions, people of color, ethnic minorities, indigenous peoples, religious minorities, migrants, people of a lower socioeconomic status, lesbian, gay, bisexual, trans, queer+ (LGBTQ+) folks, and women.[2]

Ally/Allyship

In the context of social justice, ally in its simplest form is defined as a person who supports the rights of a minority or marginalized group without being a member of it.[3] The ally definition typically recognizes that an ally is in a place of privilege and will use that advantaged position to actively support people from marginalized groups.[4] Ally is a

[a] Department of Veterinary Clinical Science, University of Surrey, UK; [b] British Veterinary Ethnicity & Diversity Society; [c] Affinity Futures Consultancy Ltd
* Corresponding author.
E-mail address: Bveds2016@gmail.com
Twitter: @issarobson (I.R.)

Vet Clin Small Anim 54 (2024) 911–924
https://doi.org/10.1016/j.cvsm.2024.07.016
0195-5616/24/© 2024 Elsevier Inc. All rights reserved, including those for text and data mining, AI training, and similar technologies.

verb, not a title. It is through consistent actions, practiced even when it is personally or professionally inconvenient, that the people you wish to support will identify you as a genuine ally.

Advocate/Accomplice

For some, the terms ally and allyship have failed to encourage the behaviors and activities that are desired in tackling inequality and terminology around allyship is currently changing. There does not seem to be a clear consensus about the specific definition of advocate or accomplice.[5–8] Activities carried out by advocates and accomplices involve greater risks (personal and professional). Advocates and accomplices go beyond interpersonal allyship, to disrupt structural disadvantage within organizations and society.[9]

The emphasis on privilege in many definitions of the words ally and advocate sets up allyship as charitable acts for the less privileged. When allies are cast as saviors, the relationship dynamics between the marginalized people they seek to support can be seen as patronizing. Accomplices realize that societal inequality affects us all and that this is not someone else's struggle they are "helping out" in. Therefore, dismantling inequity becomes a shared responsibility for accomplices.[10]

Rather than defining terms, this article will focus on the allyship journey itself, key allyship activities and criticisms.[11]

INTRODUCTION
Why is Allyship Important in the Veterinary Sector?

Organizations that want to improve their diversity and inclusion culture should consider developing allyship training programs and promoting allyship values.[12] Alongside the financial benefits of diversity and inclusion,[13] organizations with strong inclusion and belonging cultures see employees report 56% higher job performance, 75% less likely to take a sick day, 50% less likely to leave, and more likely to recommend their organizations as great places to work.[14,15] Something to consider for an industry struggling to recruit and retain its veterinary workforce globally.[16–18]

It takes courage for most people to speak up in the face of a discriminatory event. Encouraging teams to learn allyship skills and empowering staff with the confidence to advocate for others consequently means learning to advocate for themselves, including in clinical matters. Workplaces where employees feel safe to speak up generally provide safer outcomes for patients.[19,20] Allyship can be used as a tool to foster inclusive workplaces where incivilities in any form are not tolerated.

Inclusive workplaces should work for everyone, not just those with marginalized identities. Knowledge of equality law and good workplace process is protective for all employees. Looking at the current and future demographics of the profession,[21–23] the numbers of us who hold at least one or more marginalized, or minority identity, account for the majority of the workforce.

DISCUSSION
The Allyship Journey

> Like how you commit to lifelong learning in veterinary medicine, allyship requires you to commit to lifelong learning about racism, sexism, homophobia, ableism and other forms of oppression.
> —Dr Lisa Greenhill.[24]

The transition to ally, advocate, or accomplice is not going to happen overnight, it takes time to build your knowledge, experience, resilience, and skills.[25] Medical professionals should not be unfamiliar with a lifelong learning approach to acquiring the skills and personal development required for allyship.[26] Allyship turns good intentions and a desire to support marginalized communities into consistent commitments and actions that challenge inequity. In this article, we will discuss 3 key allyship activities that lay foundations for sustainable cross-community allyship: self-education, emotional self-regulation, and developing self-confidence to challenge inappropriate behaviors.[12,27,28]

Allyship Self-education

Continuous self-education is one of the most fundamental activities that allies will engage with. Learning should be independently driven without an overreliance on those you personally know from marginalized communities. Allyship activities for different marginalized communities will vary and further exploration of the literature is encouraged.

Expecting people from marginalized communities to educate you, on your schedule, phrased in a way to your liking and uncompensated for, in what can be an emotionally draining experience, could be seen as entitled. Even for the busiest of veterinary professionals, we have more audiobooks, blogs, podcasts, TV programming, Internet platforms than ever before. Many of our colleagues have been sharing their lived experiences of discrimination in our own profession for decades, we cannot now explain our knowledge gaps from a primary lack of resources. To assist in answering the question "What can I do?" **Table 1** provides a list of allyship topics to reflect on, action or practice.

Emotional Self-regulation for Challenging Conversations

When we avoid difficult conversations, we trade short term discomfort for long term dysfunction

—*Peter Bromberg*

The allyship journey can bring up difficult emotions, and it is important to point out that discomfort when discussing discrimination is likely to pass with time and practice. Being uncomfortable is a normal phase given the social conditioning around these taboo subjects.[33,34] Pushing ourselves out of our comfort zones, sitting with discomfort should be familiar territory for all former veterinary students. If we can view discomfort as a sign of potential growth, we have a powerful antidote to defensiveness reactions that stop us from having open and honest dialogs. If strong emotional reactions continue to block you from starting an allyship journey, you may find the suggested strategies to deal with difficult emotions in **Table 2** helpful.

Many see themselves as powerless to influence their environment and become overwhelmed by the scale of work needed to fight inequalities in our society. The effort required to undertake an allyship journey may seem daunting, but it also offers a wealth of personal growth and sense of integrity. Typically, we do always have some ability to address discriminatory behaviors within our own spheres of influence, even if that is only family, friends, and coworkers.

In a profession that is already prone to burnout, sustainable allyship practice should utilize supportive systems to protect mental health. Connecting with likeminded individuals and networks combats feelings of isolation and brings about a sense of solidarity and of being a part of a committed community working toward common goals.

The work will not be done all at once, it is a lifelong process. The realization that this is an intergenerational relay race, rather than a sprint, may help you to focus on the immediate tasks you have at hand.

Table 1
Allyship topics to reflect on, action, or practice

Foundational	Continuation
Allyship activities become a consistent habit practiced daily	Allyship becomes a practice influencing all your interactions and activities
Acknowledgment and understanding of the inequity, challenges, and barriers faced by marginalized groups	Awareness of how oppressive systems operate in society to marginalize communities
Independently seek out relevant information. Seek help from marginalized communities appropriately	Habitual knowledge seeking behavior, involving expanding social circles, reading lists, listening, and watching diverse social media feeds, created by marginalized people
Acknowledge the limitations of a single voice or view being representative of an entire marginalized community. Awareness of the risks of confirmation bias when seeking out sources	Seeking a breadth and depth of sources. Listening to a range of different lived experiences. Development of critical thinking and reasoning skills to apply in nuanced situations
Understanding basic terminology used in DEI work.[4,28,29]	Exploration of concepts frequently discussed in social justice and DEI work
Understand the differnt ways discrimination and bias manifests on an interpersonal level, for example, covert micro and macro agressions aswell as overt discrimination.	Understand how discrimination manifests structurally in society, institutions, and organizations. Exploration of the structural and systemic nature of oppression
Learning to challenge inappropriate and discriminatory behavior	Learning to challenge systems that perpetuate inequality, disrupting the status quo
Developing emotional resilience. Learning to sit with discomfort about challenging topics	Developing emotional resilience to sustainably engage in allyship activities
Confidence to engage publicly in challenging dialogs	Confidence to initiate, lead, and facilitate challenging discussions
Continue educational discussions within your own sphere of influence and social circles	Encourage and support others undertaking self-educating behaviors. Share and signpost to useful resources
Learning to make mistakes and give good apologies[30] Committing to do better next time	Learning from previous mistakes, with expectations of making entirely new ones
Learning how to take feedback about your behavior without defensiveness. Acting on feedback you receive	Seek out and create opportunities for safe dialogs where you can receive feedback[30]
Learning to give feedback about inappropriate behavior to prevent repeat incidents and escalation of poor behaviour	Understanding the range of responses to feedback and remaining compassionate about the receiver's ability to improve
Reflecting on past and present actions and unlearning behaviors that are harmful to others	Reflection on past and present actions that contribute to systemic inequalities. Identifying ways to change behavior
Understanding how you move through society is not the same as for marginalized people. Identifying your own positions of privilege	Learning to see the world through multiple simultaneous lenses of oppression. Considering the differences and similarities

(*continued on next page*)

Table 1 (continued)	
Foundational	**Continuation**
Reflecting on and challenging your own assumptions, beliefs, attitudes, and unconscious bias.[30]	Understanding ways in which implicit biases shape our perceptions and understandings of ourselves and others and the society we live in
Exploration of the historical inequality and injustice. Why individuals and society may hold the beliefs about marginalized groups that it does	Awareness of the link between past and present-day inequalities. Exploration of historical and current resistance movements
Developing a multilens approach to allyship activities. Awareness of processes that pit marginalized group against each other	Developing an intersectional approach to allyship. Bearing in mind the intersections of oppression, overlapping struggles, and common interests of different marginalized groups
Know your professional code of conduct in relation to discrimination[31,32]	Remind and encourage colleagues and students to uphold the professional code of conduct.
Know your workplace rights and equality laws	Understand the value of joining a union

Building the Self-confidence to Call Out Inappropriate Behaviors

"When you witness discrimination, don't approach the victim later to offer sympathy. Give them your support in the moment."[35]

The experience of discrimination can be extremely unsettling and has mental health impacts.[36] Most people have good intentions, but in the face of discrimination fail to speak up or act on behalf of those they claim to support. Silence is not allyship. Authentic allyship is not turned on or off when it is personally and professionally inconvenient.

Developing the self-confidence to challenge inappropriate behaviors is an essential allyship skill. **Table 3** provides some strategies and tips for challenging inappropriate behavior. When colleagues challenge transgressions, it can boost feelings of inclusion for marginalized individuals posttransgression, even compared to a situation where no transgression transpired.[12]

When allies speak up, they face fewer negative consequences that those from marginalized groups would themselves. When bystanders do confront discriminatory behavior, it is generally effective in changing behaviors. In addition, those that witness others confronting prejudice, are more likely to endorse antiprejudice attitudes. This type of intervention serves in setting organizational standards and norms.[37]

Cognitive dissonance is the discomfort a person can experience when their behavior does not align with their own beliefs.[38] Not speaking up in the face of inappropriate behavior is not without its own consequences for "bystanders." Inaction from bystanders feeds their own sense of helplessness, self-confidence, and has repercussion on psychological safety within the workplace.[39] The confessions of bystanders, years or even decades after an event, where they said or did nothing clearly show these incidents haunt them.

Individual Allyship in the Organizational Environment

The motivation for allies varies, and the reasons for doing allyship work may change throughout an allyship journey.[40] When allies are motivated by values, and a desire

Table 2
Helpful strategies to deal with common difficult emotions

Emotion	Strategy
Discomfort: When discussing inequality and discrimination, topics we are socially conditioned not to discuss	Discomfort is a phase that passes with time and practice. Consider discomfort instead as a sign for potential growth
Fear: Of making mistakes or being challenged about your mistakes	Approach mistakes with a growth mindset. It is natural to make mistakes in any learning journey. Do not let perfectionism hold you back. View challenges about your behavior as feedback and a request to do better in the future. Learn how to make good apologies[30]
Shame: Is the discomfort when your behavior does not align with your values. Many experience shame on the realization they have participated in harmful behaviors or actions	Avoid viewing oppression through a simple good/bad moral binary. For example, racists are bad people, and I am a good person so I cannot be racist
Embarrassment: About a lack of knowledge	It is unrealistic to know every aspect of a marginalized communities struggle. Approach knowledge acquisition with a growth mindset. Curiosity and humility are helpful in your discussions about incomplete knowledge and experience gaps. Once you have identified knowledge gaps, use them as a guide for your next steps
Overwhelm/helplessness	Reflect on and address what is within your own spheres of influence. When you are overwhelmed, focus on tasks and activities that suit your skill sets
Guilt: From the realization that you have benefited from unequitable systems or hold forms of privilege others do not	Privilege is probably better viewed as simply the absence of barriers. It can be disconcerting to find that the way you navigate the world is not the same for everyone. Use this knowledge to identify, mitigate, or remove barriers for marginalized groups where you can

to address violations of universal principles of justice and rights, they are more likely to have thought about the systemic and structural nature of how oppression operates.[41]

When an allyship journey leads to examining our own organizational policies and practices, it can be helpful to think also about the different types of actions and roles needed to bring about change. **Table 4** provides a list of allyship actions and practice that can be undertaken in organizational environments.

When considering how you can effectively bring about changes within your own organization, it is worth playing to your strengths and what is in your influence. Several authors have outlined distinct roles allies can explore, and further reading is again encouraged.[41-43]

- *Organizers* help groups achieve specific goals, committed organizers or administrators boost the sustainability of a campaign by sharing the workload.

Table 3
Strategies and tips for challenging inappropriate behavior

Strategies and Tips	Advice and Examples
Take a moment to think. Acknowledge that in the moment you will have a physical (adrenaline) and emotional response	It is difficult to think on the spot in these circumstances. Give yourself a moment to take a few deep breathed and formulate your thoughts
What stock phrases have you prepared? Life will provide you plenty of opportunities to practice. Find a stock phrase that fits your something that you will remember and use	If in doubt say *no*. No is a small word that states what your position is clearly. It also gives you some time take a breath and formulate your thoughts • No! That's not ok • That is not appropriate in the workplace • You will not talk like that in front on me
Tips for people who conflict adverse You will have opportunities to practice and grow in confidence. Find a stock phrase that fits your personality	Instead of viewing speaking up as a challenge, view it as simply stating how you feel • I am uncomfortable with this conversation • I don't feel that way • I don't agree Practice will help grow your confidence
Vocalize your values and protect your boundaries	Explain where you stand and what will happen if your boundaries are transgressed • If I hear inappropriate language, I will challenge it • If you continue to speak that way around me, you will have to leave
Tips to avoid "debates" Challenging inappropriate behavior does not need to lead to a lengthy conversation. In the moment, it may not be an appropriate time or place to hold a discussion. You might not have the mental energy or the right words to deal with explaining why something is problematic	Decline attempts to be drawn into a long conversation in the moment • I don't want to discuss this anymore • We can talk about this later, let's get on with the job • State where you stand and leave the room
Provide back up Adding your support can dramatically change the power dynamics of the situation	If you aren't the first person to speak up, make sure to provide that person with timely and public support • I agree with everything "x" has just said • Yeah, that's not appropriate
Your body language speak volumes Use it to indicate where you stand on an issue. Body language will encourage others present to speak up	• Shake your head in disagreement • Raising your hand up to protest • Catching someone's eye in the room and mouth "what?" • Go and stand next to the person who is actively challenging
A behavior doesn't sit quite right	Point out the interaction that has caused discomfort. Ask clarifying questions • Something about that feels uncomfortable • What did you mean by that? • Did you mean to make that awkward?

(continued on next page)

Table 3 (continued)	
Strategies and Tips	**Advice and Examples**
Addressing a genuine misstep/speech	Clarify what they are trying to say and then role model the correct phrasing. Provide feedback and signpost to learning resources if appropriate. Check they understand why it was inappropriate
Interrupt an uncomfortable interaction Conversations can quickly deteriorate; you may notice a suboptimal conversation making someone feel uncomfortable Provide a way for the conversation to end	Provide an opportunity for the person to escape an awkward conversation • Do you have a moment? • Can I interrupt, could you help me with this? Follow up with both parties to acknowledge that the conversation was uncomfortable. Provide feedback about why the behavior was inappropriate
Missed the moment? You didn't speak up in the moment Make sure you engage in mitigating actions after the fact	Instead of beating yourself up, reflect on what you need to do better in similar situations in the moment Follow up with both parties to acknowledge that the conversation was inappropriate. Provide feedback about why the behavior was inappropriate
Keep it professional Challenging discriminatory behavior is professional conduct[31,32]	How you challenge and the language you use will be judged by you. Keep in mind your organizations rules regarding professional conduct. Effective challenges can be made without raised voices or swearing

- *Scholars and educators* who learn about key issues facing marginalized communities, collate and communicate resources assisting other colleagues in their own learning.
- *Builders and reformers* create or change organizational policies, processes, and practices. In collective action, being good at cutting through organizational red tape can expedite change enormously.
- *Upstanders, sponsors, and confidants* are roles that offer direct support to people from marginalized groups.
- *Amplifiers, champions, and advocates* promote the inclusion of marginalized voices and groups at key events and in decision-making processes. In these high-profile roles, it is important that words are also backed up by effective actions.
- *Strategists and backers* are those who make decisions that direct, resource, support, and add legitimacy to change movements.

Allyship for Organizations

It's about creating the conditions for a climate and a culture ... where people feel comfortable to bring forth issues or concerns they may have, because that more than anything, is going to be what mitigates the potential risks that practice owners might have as it relates to discrimination

—*Julius Rhodes*[44]

In the UK, several large discrimination surveys have taken place; one of the UK vet students revealed that 29% of students had experienced discrimination and 36% had

Table 4
Allyship actions and practice in organizational environments

Foundational	Continuation
Action even in the face of professional or personal inconvenience	Action even in the face of professional risk or personal physical safety
Noticing practices, structures, and systems that perpetuate discrimination, create obstacles and inequitable outcomes	Openly challenging the status quo and campaigning for changes to systems which perpetuate bias, exclusion, and inequity
Championing marginalized people and voices	Consistent support of marginalized groups and all their activities, not just positive celebration events
Communicating your values publicly and consistently to your colleagues	Being unafraid to express public support and calling attention to a perspective or causes to the wider organization or profession
Noticing who is not able to participate in important conversations and decisions, meetings and events. Advocate for people not in the room	Ensuring that going forward there is a process to include important perspectives in the conversation
Learning the balance between speaking in support of rather than speaking for marginalized communities	Developing mechanisms to ensure marginalized voices are heard and have a platform to speak directly to the organization or profession
Support, mentor, coach, and champion marginalized individuals	Ensure mechanisms of support, mentoring and empowerment are accessible to marginalized groups
Become a safe confidant for individuals from marginalized groups through active listening	Ask affinity groups, within the profession or your own organization, how you can support them
Seek feedback about relevant issues you can influence from marginalize communities	Build a reputation of being safe person to talk to about issues, who acts, and communicates clearly throughout the process
Request organizational discrimination processes and policies are regularly communicated	Ensure that the process is fully transparent and followed Understand and challenge reporting protocols which are unsafe and ineffective
Ensure all have basic equality law, DEI training	Regular facilitated discussions within teams around issues of inclusivity. Teams have pre-emptive discussions about how to deal with all types of discriminatory incidents
Role model what inclusive leadership looks like. Signal what is not acceptable to you and what you will not let slide	Make sure those you directly are responsible for uphold your standards and creating inclusive cultures
Use your knowledge of organizational protocols to cut through red tape	Create systems where activities by marginalized groups are assisted and facilitated in a timely way by organization processes

witnessed discrimination on placement.[45] The other survey of veterinary professionals found 24% of respondents had experienced or witnessed discrimination in the last 12 months.[46] When organizations neglect to empower their staff with the tools and mechanisms to address inappropriate behavior, they undermine all other diversity, equity, and inclusion (DEI) efforts.[47]

While interpersonal barriers to allyship clearly exist, when barriers preventing allyship are explored, organizational factors (lack of training, time, resources, power, and resistance) are the most frequently cited themes.[47] If organizations can understand these barriers and address them, they are more likely to be successful in their existing and future DEI initiatives. **Table 5** outlines organizational DEI initiatives that can be enhanced through allyship activities and cultures.

Further Critiques of Allyship

If you have come here to help me, you're wasting your time. If you have come because your liberation is bound up in mine, then let us work together
—*Dr Lilla Watson.*

Further critiques of allyship warn against performative allyship, where allyship becomes merely a set of behaviors you learn to gain the moral high ground, rather than leading to effective change. Performative allyship is superficial and performed only when doing so provides accolades or personal gain.

Some question where inclusion of the marginalized into capitalist institutions and structures is really where our collective liberation lies. As the business case for diversity and inclusion gains momentum, so has the "ally industrial complex," a situation where careers, profit, and prestige are built off exploitation of the struggles of the marginalized.[48]

Allyship as charity is acting on behalf of someone else rather than yourself, and the strong emphasis in allyship on identity and privilege may reinforce the hierarchical

Table 5
Organizational allyship activities

Foundational	Continuation
Having DEI champions, roles or committee	Those that champion DEI are adequately trained, compensated (financial and time recognition) and can instigate change
Having an antidiscrimination policy or DEI statement	Clear, regular communication of values and policies throughout the veterinary organizational structure
Anonymous culture survey or feedback system (including students on placement)	Provision of psychologically safe and effective pathways for feedback in real time
DEI resources, allyship and antidiscrimination training for all staff	Regularly facilitated discussions within teams around issues of inclusivity
Decisive action taken when there is an incident	Reflection on what preventative actions could have been taken to avoid this situation. Proactive facilitated workplace discussions about discrimination
Leadership signals DEI is a core value of the organization	Management receives feedback on their inclusive leadership as part of their performance evaluations
Marginalized staff can seek support from a DEI champion	Building coalitions and support networks for communities
Creating events and celebrations for marginalized groups	Marginalized groups are invited work strategically within your organization on issues that affect them daily
Organizations expose inequitable policies and practices	Organizations effectively mitigate or change inequitable policies and practices

systems that it is supposed to be disrupting. There is now a call to move toward collaboration and coalition. Allyship as solidarity is the understanding we have a shared responsibility and will benefit from a more equal society.[49]

SUMMARY

- The practice of allyship distinguishes itself from passive forms of support for marginalized communities and those engaging in ad hoc supportive actions, particularly only when convenient or to make one look good.
- The distinctions made among ally, advocate, and accomplice should primarily encourage reflection on more progressive and strategic actions to challenge inequalities in solidarity with one another.
- Foundational allyship skills include becoming an independent learner, learning to regulate the difficult emotions which arise discussing inequity and building self-confidence to stand up to discriminatory and inappropriate behaviors.
- Allyship should not be seen as only benefiting marginalized groups. Working collectively to protect each other from discrimination and upholding each other values creates inclusive workplaces that benefit us all and lead to better patient outcomes.

CLINICS CARE POINTS

- Allyship is a tool that can help foster inclusive workplaces, where individuals feel empowered to speak out resulting in better patient care outcomes.
- Allyship can be seen as the continuous practice and activities of a person who supports the rights of a minority or marginalized group without being a member of that group.

DISCLOSURE

I. Robson is a Director of Affinity Futures Consultancy Ltd.

REFERENCES

1. Day J. What does marginalize mean: definition, examples, characteristics of the phenomenon, liberties.eu. 2022. Available at: https://www.liberties.eu/en/stories/marginalize/44083. Accessed March 30, 2024.
2. Vasas EB. Examining the margins: a concept analysis of marginalization. Adv Nurs Sci 2005;28(3):194–202. Available at: https://pubmed.ncbi.nlm.nih.gov/16106149/. Accessed March 30, 2024.
3. Oxford english dictionary, s.v. "allyship (n)". 2023. https://doi.org/10.1093/OED/2497869425. Accessed March 31, 2024.
4. Lamont A. The guide to allyship. 2021. Available at: https://guidetoallyship.com/#what-is-an-ally. Accessed March 30, 2024.
5. Jackson W. Don't be an ally, be an accomplice, medium. 2019. Available at: https://forge.medium.com/dont-be-an-ally-be-an-accomplice-437869756ab5. Accessed March 31, 2024.
6. Schafranek BA. What's the difference between an ally and accomplice? YWCA. 2021. Available at: https://www.ywcaworks.org/blogs/ywca/tue-12212021-1103/whats-difference-between-ally-and-accomplice. Accessed March 31, 2024.

7. Osler J. Moving from actor > Ally > accomplice, white accomplices. 2024. Available at: https://www.whiteaccomplices.org/. Accessed March 30, 2024.

8. Paul J. I need an accomplice, not an ally, ColorBloq.org. 2017. Available at: https://www.colorbloq.org/article/i-need-an-accomplice-not-an-ally. Accessed March 30, 2024.

9. Suyemoto KL, Hochman AL, Donovan RA, et al. Becoming and fostering allies and accomplices through authentic relationships: choosing justice over comfort. Res Hum Dev 2021;18(1-2):1–28.

10. Wilkinson RD, Pickett K. The spirit level: why more equal societies almost always do better. United Kingdom: Allen Lane/Penguin Group Bloomsbury Publishing; 2009.

11. Ponder C. Ally. advocate. warrior - why terms are irrelevant. 2018. Available at: https://medium.com/@coreytponder/ally-advocate-warrior-why-terms-are-irrelevant-6fed031fb8cf. Accessed March 30, 2024.

12. Salter NP, Migliaccio L. Allyship as a diversity and inclusion tool in the workplace. In: Diversity within Diversity Management (Advanced Series in Management)vol. 22. Emerald Publishing Limited, Leeds; 2019. p. 131–52.

13. Dixon-Fyle S., Dolan K., Hunt V., et al., Diversity wins: how inclusion matters, 2020, McKinsey & Company, Available at: https://www.mckinsey.com/featured-insights/diversity-and-inclusion/diversity-wins-how-inclusion-matters (Accessed 31 March 2024).

14. Carr EW, Reece A, Kellerman GR, et al. The value of belonging at work. Harv Bus Rev 2019. Available at: https://hbr.org/2019/12/the-value-of-belonging-at-work. Accessed March 31, 2024.

15. Hagen JR, Weller R, Mair TS, et al. Investigation of factors affecting recruitment and retention in the UK veterinary profession. Vet Rec 2020;187:354.

16. Expanding Veterinary Medicine Capacity in Canada 2022–2032: A report from the Canadian Veterinary Medical Association Veterinary Workforce Congress 2022. CVMA 2022. Available at: https://www.canadianveterinarians.net/about-cvma/latest-news/expanding-veterinary-medicine-capacity-in-canada-2022-2032-a-report-from-the-canadian-veterinary-medical-association-veterinary-workforce-congress-2022/. Accessed March 31, 2024.

17. Stay, please - a challenge to the veterinary profession to improve employee retention (2024) AAHA.org. Available at: https://www.aaha.org/practice-resources/research-center/white-paper-form-the-path-to-increasing-retention-in-veterinary-medicine/. Accessed March 31, 2024.

18. Recruitment, retention and return in the veterinary profession: preliminary report for the RCVS Workforce Summit 2021. RCVS; 2022. Available at: https://www.rcvs.org.uk/news-and-views/publications/recruitment-retention-and-return-in-the-veterinary-profession/. Accessed March 31, 2024.

19. Umoren R, Kim S, Gray MM, et al. Interprofessional model on speaking up behaviour in healthcare professionals: a qualitative study. BMJ Leader 2022;6:15–9.

20. Lewis C. The impact of interprofessional incivility on medical performance, service and patient care: a systematic review. Future Healthc J 2023;10(1):69–77.

21. AAVMC Annual Data Report 2022-2023 (2023) AAVMC.org. Available at: https://www.aavmc.org/wp-content/uploads/2023/09/2023-AAVMC-Annual-Data-Report-September23.pdf. Accessed March 31, 2024.

22. The 2019 Survey of the Veterinary Profession: A report for the Royal College of Veterinary Surgeons. 2020. Available at: https://www.rcvs.org.uk/news-and-views/publications/the-2019-survey-of-the-veterinary-profession/. Accessed March 31, 2024.

23. Kendall T. Diversity and changing demographics: How they will affect veterinary medicine. J Vet Med Educ 2004;31:406–8.

24. Greenhill L. How to be an ally. Today's Veterinary Business 2020. Available at: https://todaysveterinarybusiness.com/how-to-be-an-ally/. Accessed March 31, 2024.

25. Reid N. The good ally: a guided anti-racism journey from bystander to change-maker. London: HQ; 2022.

26. Ellis D. Bound together: allyship in the art of medicine. Ann Surg 2021;274(2): e187–8. PMID: 33856369.

27. Evans NJ, Assadi JL, Herriott TK. Encouraging the development of disability allies. N Dir Student Serv 2005;2005:67–79.

28. AAVMC Diversity, equity & inclusion glossary (2023) AAVMC.org. Available at: https://www.aavmc.org/wp-content/uploads/2021/08/Monograph-DEI-Glossary-01.pdf. Accessed March 31, 2024.

29. Odunayo A, Ng ZY. Valuing diversity in the team. Vet Clin North Am Small Anim Pract 2021;51(5):1009–40.

30. Ellevate. For allies: how to build emotional resilience for challenging conversations about race. Forbes; 2020. Available at: https://www.forbes.com/sites/ellevate/2020/09/15/for-allies-how-to-build-emotional-resilience-for-challenging-conversations-about-race/?sh=69d279dc74ca. Accessed March 30, 2024.

31. Principles of Veterinary Medical Ethics of the AVMA. American Veterinary Medical Association; 2023. Available at: https://www.avma.org/resources-tools/avma-policies/principles-veterinary-medical-ethics-avma#:~:text=As%20health%20professionals%20seeking%20to,of%20educational%2C%20training%2C%20and%20employment. Accessed March 31, 2024.

32. RCVS Code of professional conduct for Veterinary Surgeons. Section 17.5 Veterinary teams and leaders (2023) Professionals. Available at: https://www.rcvs.org.uk/setting-standards/advice-and-guidance/code-of-professional-conduct-for-veterinary-surgeons/supporting-guidance/veterinary-team-and-business/. Accessed March 31, 2024.

33. Tatum BD. Talking about race, learning about racism: the application of racial identity development theory in the classroom. Harv Educ Rev 1992;62(1):1–24. Available at: https://equity.ucla.edu/wp-content/uploads/2017/01/Tatum-Talking-About-Race.pdf.

34. DiAngelo R. White fragility why it's so hard for white people to talk about racism. Allen Lane; 2019.

35. Melaku TM, Beeman A, Smith DG, et al. Be a better ally., Harvard Business Review. 2020. Available at: https://hbr.org/2020/11/be-a-better-ally. Accessed March 30, 2024.

36. Partheeban N, Crossley BV. Experiences of racism and its impacts on mental wellbeing in Black, Asian and Minority Ethnic people working and studying in the UK veterinary sector. (MMI Research Symposium Report 2022). 2022. Available at: https://www.rcvs.org.uk/news-and-views/publications/mind-matters-research-symposium-november-2021-report/. Accessed March 30, 2024.

37. Warren M, Sekhon T, Waldrop R. Highlighting Strengths in response to discrimination: developing and testing an allyship positive psychology intervention. International J Wellbeing 2022;12:21–41.

38. Crespo M. Cognitive dissonance: analysis of the theory. Themis: Research J Justice Studies Forensic Science 2023;11(8). Available at: https://scholarworks.sjsu.edu/themis/vol11/iss1/8.

39. Russell GM. Motives of heterosexual allies in collective action for equality. J Soc Issues 2011;67:376–93.
40. Russell GM, Bohan JS. Institutional allyship for LGBT equality: underlying processes and potentials for change. J Soc Issues 2016;72:335–54.
41. Zheng L. Dei deconstructed your no-nonsense guide to doing the work and doing it right. Oakland (CA): Berrett-Koehler Publishers, Inc; 2023.
42. Catlin K. Belonging in healthcare: the better allies. Approach to creating more inclusive workplaces. Better Allies Press; 2022.
43. Catlin K. Better allies. Better Allies Press; 2021.
44. Rumple S. The scourge of discrimination, today's veterinary business. 2019. Available at: https://todaysveterinarybusiness.com/the-scourge-of-discrimination/. Accessed April 1, 2024.
45. Summers OS, Medcalf R, Hubbard KA, et al. A cross-sectional study examining perceptions of discriminatory behaviors experienced and witnessed by veterinary students undertaking clinical extra-mural studies. Front Vet Sci 2023;10. https://doi.org/10.3389/fvets.2023.940836.
46. BVA discrimination in the Veterinary Profession Statistics 2021. 2021. Available at: https://www.bva.co.uk/media/4393/bva-discrimination-stats-2021.pdf. Accessed March 31, 2024.
47. Warren M.A., Warren M.T., Bock H., et al., "If you want to be an ally, what is stopping you?" Mapping the landscape of intrapersonal, interpersonal, and contextual barriers to allyship in the workplace using ecological systems theory. 2022. Available at: https://doi.org/10.31234/osf.io/py3m5. (Accessed 31 March 2024), 2022.
48. Rudy. Accomplices not allies: abolishing the ally industrial complex, indigenous action media. 2014. Available at: https://www.indigenousaction.org/accomplices-not-allies-abolishing-the-ally-industrial-complex/. Accessed March 30, 2024.
49. Anon. From charity to solidarity: a critique of ally politics. In: Milstein C, editor. Taking sides revolutionary solidarity and the poverty of liberalism. AK Press; 2015.

One Profession, Multiple Identities
On the Implications of Intersectionality in Veterinary Medicine

Monae Roberts, MEd, MA

KEYWORDS

- Intersectionality • Diversity • Equity • Inclusion

KEY POINTS

- While strides have been made, veterinary medicine can benefit from an intersectional approach to diversity, equity, and inclusion.
- We need access to intersectional data to better understand the disparities that exist within veterinary medicine to make a more significant impact.
- Discrimination is still quite common in the United States, despite decades of policy changes and implementation of DEI practices.

INTRODUCTION

It is not standard practice for an author to speak about one's own experience or break the fourth wall to speak more directly to its audience but that is what I have decided to do. My lived experience as a Black, queer, trans-person was critical in me writing this article. It is because of this lived experience that I seek to understand the ways in which our society (the United States) perpetuates oppression and circumvents accountability. It is a peculiar situation to write to address the ways your communities have been marginalized, and systematically dehumanized, to put your life on display in an effort to be truly seen and rehumanized. To be truly seen is to be humanized, because if we all were to truly see one another, and see ourselves in the other we would struggle to dehumanize all of humanity.

It is also peculiar that a field driven by the desire to care for living creatures would not also be driven to create more equitable and inclusive spaces within. The conundrum faced by marginalized communities is that we are expected to thrive in the same systems even though these systems were not created to be inclusive of our communities. Then when we fail they can say that we are somehow deficient. It is indeed a cruel sort of torture, and it is the backdrop of our everyday lived experience.

UC Davis School of Veterinary Medicine, 944 Garrod Drive, Davis, CA 95616, USA
E-mail address: dmroberts@ucdavis.edu

Vet Clin Small Anim 54 (2024) 925–933
https://doi.org/10.1016/j.cvsm.2024.08.002   **vetsmall.theclinics.com**
0195-5616/24/© 2024 Elsevier Inc. All rights reserved, including those for text and data mining, AI training, and similar technologies.

DIVERSITY, EQUITY, AND INCLUSION ISSUES AND DISCRIMINATION

It is a well-known fact in veterinary medicine that the field has struggled to diversify the profession and is one of the most homogenous careers in the United States. In fact, a 2013 article published in *the Atlantic* identified veterinary medicine as the whitest profession in America.[1] Devastating events such as the COVID-19 epidemic and the myriad high-profile police brutality cases of the last 5 years have caused a cultural shift across the country, with sectors from commerce to housing and the medical and mental health fields taking a much-needed look at how marginalized groups are represented and served in their respective professional communities. What researchers have found in areas from academic testing and higher education admissions to the job market and patient care is that structural racism is alive and well in the United States as well as other western countries.[2–5]

A 2023 study conducted by Quillian & Lee examined trends in hiring discrimination in 6 western countries, including Canada, the United States, and the Netherlands, and found that, despite comparing data from as early as 1969 to modern data on hiring practices up through 2017, only one country (France) showed a significant decrease in hiring discrimination.[2] And this decrease was described as declining from "very high" discrimination to "high" discrimination. Several other countries actually showed an increase in discriminatory practices against ethnic groups from the Middle East and North Africa during the 2000s, with discrimination in the Netherlands generally increasing over the course of the studied period.

In Lucey and Saguil's 2020 paper examining Medical College Admission Test (MCAT) scores among Black, white, and Latinx test takers, the researchers cite the centuries-long structural and interpersonal racism that marginalized groups have faced in education, housing, and access to publicly funded aid programs as contributing significantly to disparities in educational opportunities.[4] They found that it is not overall differences in aptitude but these prolonged inequities that lead to the gap between the test scores of the most marginalized test takers and their more privileged peers.

This discrepancy in the treatment of marginalized groups pursuing educational and work opportunities also extends to their experiences seeking care and services, with medical studies aimed at patient care finding that, despite the advances in treatments available to patients, little progress has been made in addressing the disparities in accessibility due to racial bias.[6–8] A 2024 study conducted in Canada looked at patient outcomes during the height of the COVID-19 epidemic and found that immigrant populations and racialized minorities were disproportionately hospitalized for COVID-19-related illnesses, and had higher mortality rates.[9]

A recent review of racial disparities in postpartum health care highlighted that Black people with uteruses experience higher rates of mortality and morbidity as well as decreased access to postpartum care when compared to their White counterparts. Disparities such as these are often compounded by the historical context of race and medicine in the United States, with the barbaric and inhumane history of medical experimentation on Black pregnant women often leading patients at this intersection to avoid seeking medical care or struggling to advocate for their medical needs.[10]

The existing gender pay gap is common knowledge; however, something that may not be so widely known is that it has not changed much over the last 20 years, moving from 80% to 82%.[11] Building on the discussion of the gender pay gap, a statistic that clearly illustrates the need for an intersectional approach to diversity, equity, and inclusion is the existing pay gap based on gender and race. In 2022, Paul and colleagues found that "holding two disadvantaged identities simultaneously—here, being a Black woman—is associated with a multiplicative negative effect on earnings, meaning Black women are penalized both for their race and gender but also face an additional penalty for holding these two identities simultaneously."[12] Black women's earning potential is still significantly impacted by the intersections of their race and gender, this is also true for Latinx women.

They also highlight that there is a gap in the literature about intersectional wage gap considerations. Citing that "most literature on wage gaps and labor market discrimination analyzes racial wage gaps and gender wage gaps in a way that overlooks the fact that each group may face distinctive penalties for simultaneously holding more than one socially salient identity."[12] Without adequate data and research on intersectional wage gaps, making the case for policy changes to address inequities can be more challenging than it needs to be.

The implications of hiring discrimination, health care disparities, and biased admission processes are reflected in the lack of diversity in veterinary medicine and other respected career fields. There are efforts being made to remove barriers, but change is slow. Many veterinary schools have removed the Graduate Record Examination (GRE) requirement and require unconscious bias training for the selection committee and have had some success in diversifying the student body.

More recently, the Ohio State University's College of Veterinary Medicine implemented specific practices in their admissions and orientation processes aimed at increasing diversity, equity, inclusion, and belonging (they used the acronym DEIB) in their student body. The 2022 paper outlines critical barriers to promoting DEIB, including lack of awareness regarding biases, thinking that promoting DEIB is lowering standards, and failing to understand and hold others accountable for organizational cultures and expectations.[13] To address some of these barriers in their admissions process, they required admissions reviewers to attend diversity and mitigation bias training, as well as complete at least 2 implicit associations tests.

They also began decoupling irrelevant information from applications, only providing reviewers with the minimum information necessary to make informed assessments. They increased the number of reviewers to ensure that all applications meeting the minimum GPA requirements were reviewed, and they had separate reviewers assess application files and conduct interviews, ensuring that applicants were not interviewed by any reviewer who had assessed their application file. Following in the footsteps of several other higher education institutions, the school also removed GRE scores from the application process, due to the lack of evidence that GRE scores predict student success.

These and other changes were implemented over the course of 4 admission cycles, and researchers found that by the fourth cycle, historically underrepresented students comprised 35% of their student population, compared to just 10.2% in the year preceding the interventions. These positive outcomes, when taken together, highlight both the failure of classical models of admissions to select a representative and well-rounded sample of students and the success of DEI practices in ensuring that the practitioners that matriculate from veterinary medicine institutions are able to support and reflect the populations they aim to serve.

A 2008 study conducted by Sommers, Warp, and Mahoney found that the mere anticipation of participation in a racially heterogeneous group caused White study participants to exhibit more thorough information processing, leading to better understanding of the reading materials assigned as part of the intervention.[14] A 2016 paper published by Tayce and colleagues outlined the addition of a 5 week Medical Spanish course to the curriculum at the Texas A&M College of Veterinary Medicine & Biomedical Sciences.[15] Over the course of the 2 year study, researchers found that students significantly improved their medical Spanish skills, and, through simulated client interactions, increased their confidence and willingness to attempt communication with Spanish-speaking patients in their native language.

INTERSECTIONALITY

Intersectionality offers a framework for addressing the complexities of systemic discrimination, suggesting we consider the interrelatedness of our lived experience, beyond binary, either/or thinking. First coined by legal scholar and civil rights activist Kimberlé Crenshaw in 1989, the term *intersectionality* has emerged as a tool for discussing and understanding the ways in which a person's identities may impact their access to and participation in society at large. Crenshaw defines intersectionality as "... a metaphor for understanding the ways that multiple forms of inequality or disadvantage sometimes compound themselves and create obstacles that often are not understood among conventional ways of thinking."[16]

As a means of mobilizing our growing understanding of social inequality into a proactive effort to combat these systemic disparities, DEI initiatives have been implemented across the helping professions, with veterinary medicine only very recently making inroads toward a more inclusive and equitable academic and professional environment. One of the barriers to change identified in the field has been its inherent focus on animal health and well-being, which has allowed for DEI themes in the training and practice of the humans providing services to remain underemphasized.[3] Despite this oversight, various research studies in the health fields have demonstrated that integrating DEI concepts into the training and practice of health-focused services creates a more inclusive and impactful environment for students, practitioners, patients, and guardians.[5,13,14,16–19]

While these efforts have helped, there is a long road ahead and much to be desired regarding more expansive approaches. Intersectionality represents possibility, and the capacity to create more intentionally inclusive, and ultimately holistic practices, putting into practice the old adage of killing two birds with one stone. There are many examples of society having a more expansive and inclusive view of experiences and situations. For example, having medications that address a variety of health conditions, interdisciplinary approaches within education, laws and court decisions, even in nature we find that very rarely do we see anything as being one dimensional or serving one purpose only.

Another concept to consider that has a similar quality is the concept of One Health. While intersectionality and One Health are different, both center on the idea that solving complex problems with a one-dimensional lens will limit how successful we can be in effectively addressing issues. You cannot separate the environment from the animal, the plants, and the people. You cannot separate gender from race, sexuality, and disability, and so forth. When you do, you run the risk of not successfully addressing the issue, much like placing a bucket under a leaky pipe that will eventually overflow.

We understand that systems and life experiences are complex, with many aspects to consider. Even when considering the best course of treatment for an animal, veterinary professionals must consider the whole animal—the size, the breed, the stage of life, genetic conditions, the environment, and so forth. So why is it that when we practice diversity, equity, and inclusion, do we tend to consider individual identities in a vacuum? Why do we collect statistics on identities of veterinary professionals but do not look at the intersectional data to gain a more nuanced understanding of the experiences of those within the margins of the margins?

We cannot ignore the serious implications for marginalized communities when we reduce their lived experience to a single identity without the nuance of intersectionality as the backdrop. "Simplistic data categories often overlook the complex, intersectional nature of inequality, causing tension with traditional data science methods."[20] It is tantamount to treating only one health issue at a time even when they are dependent on one another.

It seems as though intersectionality has one big difference between these other examples of having a more expansive and inclusive application, intersectionality specifically highlights the issues we experience in society. It forces us to look at the not so pretty side of the whole part. It is too uncomfortable to consider that some people in our society thrive at the expense of others. Intersectionality represents the equity and inclusion, the shadow side to the bright and shiny diversity. Organizations more frequently say they want diversity without considering what that diversity means. Who is included in the diversity you speak of? As more (White) women began to enter the veterinary profession one might say it was a huge win for DEI efforts, and this would only be partially true. This is not to minimize the work done previously in support of gender equality in the field; however, it is important that we do not celebrate prematurely; there is still work to be done. If your DEI practice is only inclusive of the marginalized individuals who are most adjacent to privilege, that is selective diversity without equity and inclusion. Intersectionality is the intentionality behind diversity, equity, and inclusion in DEI. Without it, you just have the illusion of diversity without equity and inclusion.

The Combahee River Collective (CRC), a Black Feminist Lesbian organization, founded by Barbara Smith in 1974, was born out of the frustration of some identities being centered over others within civil rights spaces.[21] The CRC understood that in order to address discrimination and systemic oppression it was critical to consider all forms of oppression in the larger context rather than separating out identities and trying to fight for a single identity to gain liberation. It is in the fight for individual freedom that we lose our greatest strength—being many with similar struggles. The systems that maintain oppression and domination thrive when we continue to struggle separately or seek liberation for some identities we hold while silencing other parts of ourselves.

The Combahee River Collective Statement states that if Black women were to be free it would necessitate the freedom of all other people.[22] Unfortunately, there are a substantial number of individuals in power that believe that their freedom lies in the oppression and subjugation of other communities. If energy is put into creating equity and inclusion for those who are most marginalized by a policy or practice (at the time, many of them argued this was Black women), it would by de facto also lead to the liberation of all people. So how does that work exactly? Ultimately this is about access, ensuring the greatest access possible for all parties. One example would be curb cuts at the corners of a sidewalk. Creating the curb cuts does not prevent or hinder people from walking across the street but it does also allow people using wheels to move around to also safely cross. People using wheelchairs would benefit but so would caregivers with strollers or a person riding a scooter or bike. Considering the court case in which intersectionality was first used, an equitable policy might be to hire based on skill set and expertise required for the position by removing identifying information from the hiring process, providing rubrics to stay focused on skills and experience.

A drug that can address more than one health condition is potentially more useful than a drug that only addresses one condition. Consider this in regard to multiple marginalized identities. If we create policies and practices within systems that address the oppression of multiple marginalized identities, it has the potential to have a greater impact for more people across the system. If we put energy into creating systems that remove barriers and reduce discrimination for those individuals on the margins of the margins it would not only provide greater quality of life for those people, but it would also do so for all people within the system, even those with extreme power that do not seem to need any support.

The sociocultural issues of a nation are not something that is easy to address, mainly the health implications are not recognized by everyone. You cannot find it under a microscope, or see it on a radiograph or MRI. As human beings, we have a hard time addressing the intangible. While the sociocultural issues may be intangible, their impact produces very tangible consequences for marginalized communities. Another barrier to addressing sociocultural issues is that, specifically in the United States, our culture is not a collectivist culture, rather it is one that prides itself on the individual being able to work their way to success without any support. This creates a culture of each person for themselves and reinforces the belief that the sociocultural issues are the fault of the individual rather than the responsibility of the collective. It is also false that any one person is solely responsible for their own success because we are all dependent on one another at one point or another. What use is intersectionality theory if we, as a society, believe that all things boil down to individual responsibility?

Freedom is a dependent variable; none of us is truly free until we are all free. Those with immense power within the system are not truly free because in order to maintain their power that affords them this "freedom" they must uphold the system. So they are a victim to the system they use to oppress others, although they do not realize it and it impacts them to a much lesser extent. If they decide to no longer uphold the system, the system will treat them as it treats others who go against it, whether that be intentionally or unintentionally. Our freedom is interconnected, "we are caught in an inescapable network of mutuality, tied in a single garment of destiny. Whatever affects one directly, affects all indirectly."[23] At some point, we must begin to recognize this and respond accordingly. Lilla Watson said it very plainly, "If you have come here to help me, you are wasting your time. But if you have come because your liberation is bound up with mine, then let us work together." Only when we truly believe in this mutuality and act on this belief will things begin to shift.

SUMMARY

What are the practical implications for utilizing intersectionality to support more equity and inclusion within veterinary medicine? The first application is policy development. Consider the origins of its application with the Combahee River Collective (although not directly referred to, the sentiment of what was being said in the CRC statement aligns seamlessly with intersectionality) was initially developed as a means to express the politics of the collective, that is, the way in which they make decisions. "The most general statement of our politics at the present time would be that we are actively committed to struggling against racial, sexual, heterosexual, and class oppression, and see as our particular task the development of integrated analysis and practice based upon the fact that the major systems of oppression are interlocking." Are we intersectional in our policy and our praxis? When we make decisions within the veterinary medicine sphere (although I would honestly say this applies more broadly as well) are we making sure our policies remove barriers to participation rather than add to them? This is where we should ask the question: Who might we be excluding from participating with this policy?

Another application is community engagement. It is important that we ask our-selves: who is missing from the community, who are we not serving, who is not engaging, what are the needs of our community, who is at risk of not having their needs met, and then we must ask why. Ultimately, we must be the goal and the means to achieve the goal; it is our responsibility as community to use all the tools (intersec-tionality) to co-create the society we want to live in; we are the ones we have been waiting for.

Finally, intersectionality must be used in data science, especially data pertaining to faculty, staff, and students, as well as the communities we serve. Bentley and col-leagues suggest that some data lose their capacity to address inequities because data scientists do not utilize a "more nuanced understanding of intersectionality."[20] Ultimately, intersectionality is perhaps the missing link to making huge strides in creating greater equity and developing a sense of belonging within veterinary med-icine. As stated earlier, when we do not have intersectional data and research, we are limiting the possibilities of our equity work. To put it boldly, intersectionality "is a significant forum for investigating and transforming relationships between people, places and institutions, toward human rights, reduced inequality and social justice."[24]

I began this article inviting you to see me and consider the peculiar state of exis-tence many marginalized communities live through on a daily basis. To close, I want to invite you to see yourself, wholly and extensively, through and through. See the parts of yourself that maybe you have been taught to hide, or that you feel shame around. I want to invite you to see the connection and understand that we all have those parts and in continuing to hide we disempower ourselves and give power to the systems that seek to maintain oppression. So instead, I invite you to choose inte-gration, choose to bring forth all your parts and decide how you will show up moving forward. Who will you be? Will you interrogate each part to determine whether it is true to you, or simply an abstraction you have been conditioned to believe? Will you be whole? Will you invite others to be whole? Will you create space for all the parts of the whole? Will you choose liberation for all over comfort and complacency?

CLINICS CARE POINTS

- Consider how your clients, especially those with more marginalized and hidden identities, might experience your practice.

- What systems and practices do you have in place that create a greater sense of inclusion in your clinic?.

- It is important that clients feel that they can bring their full selves into the clinic to receive care for their animals.

- This practice of more expansive inclusion can allow for a better understanding of how to care for the patient when considering the client's capacity and priorities.

- The work of becoming more inclusive is work that takes place on and off the clock.

- It is a commitment to expanding the internal culture of yourself, to show up in the clinic focused on being more inclusive each day.

DISCLOSURE

The author has nothing to disclose.

REFERENCES

1. Noel NL, Abrams J, Mudafort ER, et al. Study protocol for the implementation of Centering Patients with Fibroids, a novel group education and empowerment program for patients with symptomatic uterine fibroids. Reprod Health 2024;21(1): 41. PMID: 38561795; PMCID: PMC10983732.
2. Berger JT, Miller R, Ethnocentrism D. Racism, and the misuse of culture in US medical professional organizations: the case of hospice and palliative care. J Gen Intern Med 2024;39:847–50.
3. Taha Asma. Belonging, justice, and accessibility in pediatric health care. J Pediatr Health Care 2024;38(Issue 2):P107–8.
4. Agarwal AK, Gonzales RE, Sagan C, et al. Perspectives of black patients on racism within emergency care. JAMA Health Forum 2024;5(3):e240046.
5. Bentley C, Muyoya C, Vannini S, et al. Intersectional approaches to data: the importance of an articulation mindset for intersectional data science. Big Data & Society 2023;10(2).
6. Timmenga FSL, Jansen W, Turner PV, et al. Mental well-being and diversity, equity, and inclusiveness in the veterinary profession: pathways to a more resilient profession. Front Vet Sci 2022. https://doi.org/10.3389/fvets.2022.888189. 28 July 2022 Sec. Veterinary Humanities and Social Sciences Volume 9 - 2022.
7. Silverman DM, Rosario RJ, Hernandez IA, et al. The ongoing development of strength-based approaches to people who hold systemically marginalized identities. Pers Soc Psychol Rev 2023;27(3):255–71.
8. Sommers SRW, Lindsey S, Mahoney CC. Cognitive effects of racial diversity: white individuals' information processing in heterogeneous groups. J Exp Soc Psychol 2008;44(4):1129–36.
9. Avant ND, Davis RD. Navigating and supporting marginalized identities in dominant pharmacy spaces. Innov Pharm 2018;9(4). https://doi.org/10.24926/iip.v9i4. 1033.
10. Alvarez EE, Gilles WK, Lygo-Baker S, et al. How to approach cultural humility debriefing within clinical veterinary environments. J Vet Med Educ 2021;48(3): 256–62.
11. Alvarez EE, Gilles WK, Lygo-Baker S, et al. Teaching cultural humility and implicit bias to veterinary medical students: a review and recommendation for best practices. J Vet Med Educ 2020;47(1):2–7.
12. Crenshaw K. Demarginalizing the intersection of race and sex: a black feminist critique of antidiscrimination doctrine, feminist theory, and antiracist politics. Univ Chicago Leg Forum 1989;14:538–54.
13. Milstein MS, Gilbertson MLJ, Bernstein LA, et al. Integrating the Multicultural Veterinary Medical Association actionables into diversity, equity, and inclusion curricula in United States veterinary colleges. J Am Vet Med Assoc 2022; 260(10):1145–52.
14. Combahee River collective statement. Available at: https://americanstudies.yale. edu/sites/default/files/files/Keyword%20Coalition_Readings.pdf. Accessed March 31, 2024.
15. Black history boston. Combahee river collective. Available at: https://www.boston. gov/news/black-history-boston-combahee-river-collective. Accessed March 31, 2024.
16. King. Martin luther letter from A birmingham jail. Available at: https://www.africa. upenn.edu/Articles_Gen/Letter_Birmingham.html. Accessed March 31, 2024.

17. Tayce JD, Burnham S, Mays G, et al. Developing cultural competence through the introduction of medical Spanish into the veterinary curriculum. J Vet Med Educ 2016 Winter;43(4):390–7.
18. Quillian L, Lee JJ. Trends in racial and ethnic discrimination in hiring in six Western countries. Proc Natl Acad Sci USA 2023;120(6). e2212875120.
19. Lucey CR, Saguil A. The consequences of structural racism on MCAT scores and medical school admissions: the past is prologue. Acad Med 2020 Mar;95(3): 351–6. PMID: 31425184.
20. Thompson D. The 33 whitest jobs in America the Atlantic. 2013. Available at: https://www.theatlantic.com/business/archive/2013/11/the-33-whitest-jobs-in-america/281180/. Accessed March 31, 2024.
21. Paul M, Zaw K, Darity W. Returns in the labor market: a nuanced view of penalties at the intersection of race and gender in the US. Fem Econ 2022;28(2):1–31.
22. Rishworth A, Wilson K, Adams M, et al. Landscapes of inequities, structural racism, and disease during the COVID-19 pandemic: experiences of immigrant and racialized populations in Canada. Health Place 2024;87:103214.
23. Burkhard MJ, Dawkins S, Knoblaugh SE, et al. Supporting diversity, equity, inclusion, and belonging to strengthen and position the veterinary profession for service, sustainability, excellence, and impact. J Am Vet Med Assoc 2022;260(11): 1283–90.
24. ARAGÃO C. Gender pay gap in U.S. hasn't changed much in two decades. 2023. Available at: https://www.pewresearch.org/short-reads/2023/03/01/gender-pay-gap-facts/.

Beginning with the End in Mind

Creating a Practice that Centers Equity—Part 1

Emilia Wong Gordon, DVM, DABVP (Shelter Medicine Practice)*

KEYWORDS

- Equity • Veterinary medicine • Access to care • Discrimination • Trauma-informed
- Psychological safety • Social determinants of health

KEY POINTS

- Equity seeks to ensure that every person and nonhuman animal has what they need, while acknowledging the presence of barriers arising from historical exclusion and differential access to power and resources.
- Inequities in veterinary medicine stem from broader social inequities and pose a threat to team member well-being and access to veterinary care.
- Veterinary team members who identify as part of systemically excluded groups help facilitate access to care by fostering empathy and reducing barriers for community members, but they are also at risk of experiencing workplace discrimination, trauma, and other harms.
- Human–animal families experiencing barriers to health equity due to resource disparities love their animals and are at risk of poor outcomes, including family separation.

INTRODUCTION

"Diversity is a fact. Equity is a choice. Inclusion is an action. Belonging is an outcome."[1]

Equity has many definitions (**Box 1**), but it usually means every person has what they need *and* acknowledges historical and current factors that disproportionately create barriers for some people and groups while privileging others.[2–4] Veterinary medicine has typically focused on diversity and inclusion, not equity. In a recent webinar, half the attendees were familiar with these 2 terms, but only one-third were familiar with equity.[5]

Haven Veterinary Services, Vancouver, British Columbia, Canada
* PO Box 45010 Dunbar, Vancouver, British Columbia V6S 2M8, Canada.
E-mail address: egordon@havenvetservices.ca

Vet Clin Small Anim 54 (2024) 935–958
https://doi.org/10.1016/j.cvsm.2024.07.017   vetsmall.theclinics.com

Box 1
Select published definitions of equity

1. The guarantee of fair treatment, access, opportunity, and advancement while at the same time striving to identify and eliminate barriers that have prevented the full participation of some groups. The principle of equity acknowledges that there are historically underserved and underrepresented populations and that fairness regarding these unbalanced conditions is needed to assist equality in the provision of effective opportunities to all groups."[3,6] (Definition used by the American Association of Veterinary Medical Colleges)

2. Equity refers to fairness and justice and is distinguished from equality; while equality means providing the same to all, equity requires recognizing that we do not all start from the same place because power is unevenly distributed; the process of achieving equity is ongoing, requiring us to identify and overcome uneven distribution of power as well as intentional and unintentional barriers arising from bias or structural root causes."[7,8(p135)] (Definition from The Routledge International Handbook of Human-animal Interactions and Anthrozoology)

3. Equity is the measured experience of individual, interpersonal, and organizational success and well-being across all stakeholder populations and the absence of discrimination, mistreatment, or abuse for all. Equity is achieved by eliminating structural barriers resulting from historical and present-day inequities and meeting individuals', groups', and organizations' unique needs."[4(p39)] (Workplace definition from DEI Deconstructed)

In veterinary practice, equity is important for team members and the populations they serve (clients, patients, students, and so forth). Veterinary medicine is health care: keeping animals healthy promotes physical and mental health of human caregivers.[9,10] The Center for Disease Control defines health equity as "the state in which everyone has a fair and just opportunity to attain their highest level of health. This requires ongoing societal efforts to: address historical and contemporary injustices; overcome economic, social, and other obstacles to health and health care; and eliminate preventable health disparities."[11] Building equity in veterinary practice has several layers (**Box 2**) and involves the physical environment, clinical policies and practices, and culture.

This article is the first of a two part series and will define relevant terminology, review barriers related to systemic exclusion, and describe impacts of these barriers on veterinary teams and clients/community members. The second article will explore current controversies and detail recommendations for equity in veterinary practice.

Box 2
Relevant layers of practice

1. A physical veterinary practice or other private, public, or nonprofit facility with veterinarians.[12,13]

2. The activity of clinical practice by individual practitioners and practice teams, that is, "To be professionally engaged in."[14]

3. The concept of practice as the intentional repetition of a skill or approach to gain proficiency.[14,15] In medicine, this includes learning, reflection, feedback, communication, and growth.[15]

Terminology

Definitions of commonly used terms can be found in the Glossary at the end of this article. Collective terminology used to refer to persons identifying as part of one or more groups that have been historically, persistently, or systemically excluded based on race, ethnicity, religion, gender and/or sexual identity, disability, age, and other identity traits varies.[3,16] "Systemically excluded" or "marginalized" will be used here to denote active social exclusion from mainstream norms, which often includes the presence of barriers to accessing power and resources.[3,8,16]

Additional characteristics associated with discrimination within veterinary workplaces will be discussed, including pregnancy, parenthood, neurodiversity, and speaking English with a nonnative accent. Other barriers, such as body size, socioeconomic status, addiction and recovery, and dietary needs, have not been explored in the veterinary literature[17,18] and will not be addressed.

The term "racialized" is widely used in Canada rather than "minority/minoritized," "Black, Indigenous, People of Color," or "people of color." "Racialized" is sometimes preferred as it conveys race as a social construct, shifts focus from population demographics to differential access to power, and is inclusive of multiracial people.[19–21] Along with other terms that group all non-White people together, it has been criticized for erasing differences between experiences of various racialized groups, normalizing whiteness, and not explicitly acknowledging the deeply entrenched systemic, structural, and institutional racism affecting Black and Indigenous people.[20,22,23] Current literature describing discrimination in veterinary medicine generally does not disaggregate racial data. Therefore, "racialized" will refer to all people who "do not identify as primarily White in race, ethnicity, origin, or color,"[16] with White defined as "people originating from Europe,"[24] except where a person self-identifies differently or in quotes from source material using different terminology.

BACKGROUND

When seeking to have an equity-focused practice, a good starting point is to ask

Who Is Represented? Who Has Been Systemically Excluded?

Veterinary medicine has long been recognized as a profession with a glaring lack of racial diversity (**Table 1**). For example, the number of Black veterinarians in the United States is limited and dwindling proportionally (from 2.1% in 2016 to 1.3% in 2023).[25] In Canada, demographic data for the entire veterinary profession are not available; however, the lack of diversity is thought to mirror the United States.[26,27]

In the United States, pet ownership is varied across racial and ethnic demographics. In a 2023 survey of English-speaking and Spanish-speaking adults, 62% of participants overall had pets, with pet ownership reported by 37%, 34%, 66%, and 68% of Asian, Black, Latino/Hispanic, and White respondents, respectively.[33] Pets were regarded as family by 97% of respondents across income levels, with women (57%) and participants with lower income (64%) more likely than those with mid-income (46%) or high-income (43%) to describe pets as "as much a part of their family as a human member."[33]

What Are the Historical and Present-day Inequities?[4]

There is often a relationship between being part of a systemically excluded group and experiences of discrimination as well as reduced access to financial resources (income and accumulated wealth).[34–36] The social determinants of health (SDoH) include social, political, and economic factors—such as housing, race, gender, and

Table 1
Racial/ethnic and gender breakdown of veterinary profession versus population as a whole

	US Veterinarians[a] (%)	US Veterinary Technicians[a] (%)	US Population as a whole[25] (%)	Canadian Veterinarians[b] (%)	Canadian Population as a whole[28,29] (%)
Race					
White (non-Hispanic)	90	89.8	58.9	Unknown	67.4
Black	1.3	5.7	13.6	Unknown	4.3
Hispanic/Latino	7.9	10.2	19.1	Unknown	1.6
Asian	5.9	2.5	6.3	Unknown	19.3
American Indian/Alaska Native/Native Hawaiian/Pacific Islander/Indigenous	0.2[30]	Unknown	1.6	Unknown	4.9
Multiracial	Unknown	Unknown	Unknown	Unknown	3.2
Gender					
Female	69.1	89.9	50.4	64	50.1
Male	Unknown	Unknown	Unknown	35.5	49.9
Undisclosed/unknown	Unknown	Unknown	Unknown	0.5	Unknown

[a] Data based on 87,000 veterinarians and 142,000 veterinary technicians.[31]
[b] Data from Canadian Veterinary Medical Association (voluntary association representing a subset of veterinarians in Canada).[32] There are no publicly available data for veterinary technicians in Canada.

income—with profound impacts on lives and health outcomes of companion animals and their caregivers.[37–39] Understanding the SDoH is crucial to adopting a sustainable and empowering "strengths-based" (vs "deficit-based") perspective toward equity in practice.[40,41]

Systemic and structural inequities are linked to racial wealth gaps in the United States and Canada. In the United States, for every US$1 of net worth for a White family, Asian, Black, Hispanic, and Indigenous families have 83, 6, 7, and 8 cents, respectively.[34,36] In both countries, there are resource-access gaps by gender, sexual identity, disability, and other SDoH.[28,42–47] Systemic oppression and differential access to resources directly impact veterinary clients and their animals, as well as veterinary team members.

Extensive exploration of the historical origins of current inequities affecting veterinary medicine is beyond the scope of this article. These disparities are rooted in systems deliberately established to allocate power and resources inequitably and in structures that uphold these systems by differential distribution of resources across individuals and groups.[48,49] Examples include the transatlantic slave trade, genocide of Indigenous peoples in North America, and historical legislation limiting rights of racialized people, women, and others.[4,24,49]

What Are the Barriers and Impacts that Arise from These Inequities?

Veterinary teams

Inequities that disproportionately impact people from systemically excluded groups impact veterinary teams, clients, and animals. For veterinary service providers, generational wealth is inversely proportional to student debt load. On average, Black veterinarians have US$100,000 more debt than White veterinarians.[50] Debt load and financial worries contribute to poor well-being and psychological distress, particularly in younger veterinarians.[51]

Although much of the primary literature is focused on veterinarians, burnout and psychological distress were higher among support staff than veterinarians in several studies.[51,52] Because equity-related topics discussed relate to systemic factors, it is likely that veterinary support staff experience similar barriers and impacts.

Racial and ethnic identity

"I was one of three Black women in my graduating class. Throughout our vet school career, most of our classmates used our three names interchangeably. They couldn't bother to figure out who was who."[53]

There is limited peer-reviewed literature on experiences of racialized veterinary professionals in North America, but in recent UK studies, racialized veterinary students reported discrimination, a lack of diversity, and reluctance to report/lack of confidence in reporting systems.[17,54] In a study on student placements in veterinary practices, 36% had perceived (witnessed or experienced) discrimination, with ethnicity (15.7%) second only to gender (38%).[17] Racism displayed by clients included expression of racist and xenophobic views and preferences for White veterinarians.[17]

A 2022 Ontario Veterinary Medical Association survey revealed that only 57% of racialized respondents felt "like I belong in the profession" (vs 81% of all respondents).[55] Additionally, 52% of racialized veterinarians (vs 28% nonracialized) reported experiencing discrimination in the profession.[55] In 2020, the Multicultural Veterinary Medical Association asked the veterinary sector to share experiences with racism and discrimination and collected 387 narratives over 9 days, suggesting that racism is widespread.[53]

"Tell this Ching Chong Chang vet she's wrong, I don't ever want to see her again. She shouldn't practice in this country."[56]

Racialized team members who are nonnative English speakers may experience accent discrimination, a subtle, yet often "socially acceptable" form of racism.[56] Due to an "accent hierarchy," some accents (eg, Asian) are considered less prestigious and pleasant than British or French accents.[57,58] Linguistic racism, manifesting as stereotyping, bullying, and mocking, negatively impacts mental health of international students.[59] Veterinary students who feel "less capable" of speaking English may hesitate to participate in clinical discussions, which may be perceived as a lack of knowledge and detrimentally affect future employment.[60] Immigration intersects with linguistic racism, with increasing opportunities for tension as more internationally trained vets come to North America due to structural deficiencies in training veterinarians domestically.[61,62]

Gender and sexism

"The specialized opinion of a woman with more years [of] experience and board certification was ignored for that of a man not even graduated 5 years. All the men in the room deferred to him."[17]

The veterinary profession is becoming increasingly feminized, yet gender discrimination is common.[17,63–66] In multiple surveys of veterinarians and veterinary students, gender discrimination was the most frequently reported form of discrimination (reported by 19%–38% of respondents).[17,65,66] Gender discrimination frequently intersects with other forms of discrimination, for example, racism, homophobia, and pregnancy discrimination, with racialized and lesbian, gay, bisexual, transgender, queer and intersex (LGBTI+) respondents reporting higher rates of gender discrimination.[65] Female veterinarians are less likely to consider leadership roles such as practice ownership,[67] and experiencing discrimination affects their professional aspirations.[65] This could have rippling effects, as a study on women in leadership roles found that many were motivated by a desire to enact positive change, including through mentoring.[68]

Overall, veterinarians experience more negative psychological health than the general population.[69–72] Female veterinarians are at particular risk, reporting increased psychological distress, reduced well-being, and less-favorable workplace psychosocial conditions.[69–72] Despite a persistent gender pay gap,[73] in one study 44% of hiring managers (men and women) believed women no longer face gender discrimination in the profession.[64] These managers reviewed identical performance evaluations for a veterinarian named Mark or Elizabeth, offered Mark a significantly higher salary, and considered him more competent.[64]

Pregnancy and parenting

"At an interview, a male owner told me I could never be a good vet and a good mom."[74]

Several studies of veterinarians and vet students reported challenges with pregnancy, lactation, and parenthood.[74–76] These include a lack of formal parental leave policies, inflexible schedules, delaying starting a family during training due to a lack of institutional support, guilt balancing parenthood with veterinary medicine (worse for women), and lack of spaces for pumping breastmilk.[74–76]

Additionally, 25% to 36.4% of pregnant respondents reported feeling unsafe or "unsure of their safety" at work.[74,76] In one study, 72.9% of mothers reported experiencing maternal discrimination including sexist and discriminatory comments and negative impacts on compensation and promotion/employment opportunities[74] which is double the rate for physician mothers.[77]

Sexual and gender identity

"I experienced a lot of fear surrounding people finding out that I am in a same-sex relationship, which resulted in panic attacks."[78]

Veterinarians and veterinary team members identifying as 2SLGBTQIA+ may be overrepresented compared to the general population.[79] Studies of 2SLGBTQIA+ veterinary professionals (veterinarians, registered veterinary technician [RVTs], and other team members) and students in the United States and United Kingdom reported that 35% to 45% experienced workplace difficulties due to their sexual orientation or gender identity.[78,80] The most common outcome of attempts to resolve these challenges was that they were not resolved (27%), with another 14.5% reporting resolution through changing jobs or graduating, and only 13.8% reporting resolution through "self-acceptance or acceptance from others."[78]

Veterinarians are at higher risk of suicide than the general population, with the highest risk in small animal practice (male and female veterinarians have 2.1 and 3.5 times the risk, respectively).[81] Furthermore, lesbian, gay, bisexual, transgender, queer, questioning, and asexual (LGBTQ+) veterinary professionals had an even higher lifetime risk of both suicidal ideation and attempted suicide than veterinarians as a whole.[72,80]

Age

Ageism is a widespread and socially acceptable form of discrimination,[82] affecting young and older workers, usually persons aged less than 35 years or greater than 55 years.[82–84] The belief that older workers are less valuable and productive has been described as originating from Western cultural norms that associate "aging with decline, dependency, isolation, and poverty."[85] Ageism often intersects with other discrimination, for example, sexism, ableism, and racism.[82,86]

One study of veterinary students described discrimination based on young age/perceived inexperience for those aged less than 27 years, whereas some students aged 28 to 35 years reported discrimination based on older age.[17] Other veterinary references focus mainly on older workers, detailing misconceptions about workers aged greater than 40 years as less tech savvy and productive, and more costly, despite data that productivity and job stability increase with age, whereas absenteeism and workplace accidents decrease.[85,87,88] In a clinical setting, mature practitioners contribute valuable experience and mentorship, and age diversity on a veterinary team may be valued by clients.[88]

Disability and chronic illness

There is limited research on ableism in veterinary medicine and experiences of veterinary team members with disabilities, but 15% to 20% of adults live with disabilities,[89] and work-related injuries are common in veterinary medicine.[90] In Canada and the United Kingdom, 4.5% to 8.7% of survey respondents reported disability or chronic illness; definitions varied, but usually included dyslexia and other forms of neurodiversity.[17,55,66,91] In one study, 46.7% of participants with a disability witnessed or experienced ableism-based discrimination (vs 4.6% of respondents with no reported disability); respondents mostly reported "nonphysical and/or invisible disabilities."[17] Reduced belonging and increased discrimination and feelings of being "silenced or dismissed," compared to respondents without disability were reported in Canada.[55]

People with disabilities often experience workplace discrimination and reduced compensation and employment opportunities, and they are underrepresented in health professions.[89,92] Compared to those with physical disabilities, workers with nonphysical disabilities "reported more negative experiences," perhaps due to their accommodations being regarded as less fair.[92] Conversely, those with visible disabilities were more likely to experience ableist microaggressions, with negative impacts on mental health.[93] Extrapolating from human health care, providers with disabilities likely benefit patients, because providers should represent those they serve, and those with disabilities may have more empathy for clients and patients.[89,94,95]

Neurodiversity

Although not considered a disability,[96] neurodiversity is often lumped into a "disability" category, limiting demographic information.[17,55] Neurodiversity is "the idea that people experience and interact with the world around them in many different ways; there is no one "right" way of thinking, learning, and behaving, and differences are not viewed as deficits."[97] Neurodiversity includes autism spectrum disorder (ASD)/autism spectrum conditions, attention deficit hyperactivity disorder, dyslexia, and other neurologic and developmental conditions.[97,98] Neurodivergent people are more likely to experience underemployment, unemployment, and job loss than neurotypical people.[96]

In the sole English-language study on experiences of veterinarians with ASD, autistic veterinarians had markedly reduced mental well-being and described poor psychosocial work conditions compared to other veterinarians or the workforce in general.[98] Autistic adults may be overrepresented in veterinary medicine as the profession values "autistic traits," for example, detail-oriented, problem-solving, and ability to hyperfocus.[98] Several non-peer-reviewed articles about neurodiversity in veterinary medicine describe strengths, for example, creativity, visual/spatial skills, and passion, that neurodivergent team members contribute to enhance veterinary teams.[99–102]

Religious identity

"My Sikh practice owner had to stop wearing his turban because people called him a sand n— — —."[53]

More people are Christian than any other religion, both globally and in North America.[103] Religious discrimination against people practicing minority religions has been reported in society and health care.[104] There are apparently no studies on religious discrimination in veterinary medicine. In both the United States and Canada, there have been sustained increases in anti-Semitism and Islamophobia, with sharp increases in 2023.[105,106] In a 2016 study of Sikh men in New York City, men with turbans experienced more discrimination; this was associated with physical and mental health detriments.[107]

Several US studies of Muslim physicians in human health care detailed widespread and rising experiences of workplace Islamophobia, a lack of organizational accommodation for religious practices, and negative professional impacts (including patient refusal to see Muslim providers).[108,109] Respondents also reported negative impacts on "personal well-being."[108] Religious discrimination and racial discrimination overlap, both because health care providers may have intersectional identities, and because many forms of religious discrimination inherently reflect racism.

Veterinary Clients

"If practitioners working in human-animal interactions are to support the health and wellbeing of the people and animals living in the communities we serve, we must engage in self-reflection around how systems of oppression and marginalization have played out in our own lived experience and seek to change the systems that create and perpetuate this hierarchy of oppression."[7(p124)]

The SDoH affect client and patient health outcomes, with 18% and 28% of Canadian and US households, respectively, being unable to access preventive, sick, and/or emergency care for their pet.[10,110] Access to care is not "even" across sociodemographic groups and geographic areas.[37,111] Cost is the most frequently reported barrier to accessing care; other barriers include lack of transportation, distance, limited provider availability, fear of judgment, linguistic differences, other personal limitations (eg, health), and pet-specific factors (eg, species).[10,112]

People experiencing marginalization and loss (eg, bereavement) and those who are low-income may be more attached to their pets and rely on them more for comfort than those who are not marginalized and/or high-income.[33,113,114] Individuals and families who lack generational wealth and/or struggle with challenges relating to costs of veterinary care, as well as housing and personal health, are at risk of human–animal family separation through relinquishment or economic euthanasia.[115–118]

When animal welfare and the human–animal bond are imperiled due to lack of access to veterinary care, it can cause profound trauma to those already struggling or at highest risk of social harm. The common statement "pet ownership is a privilege, not a right" is often used when an owner is struggling to access care; however, it is harmful and contravenes equity because it "legitimizes maintenance of the status quo in veterinary service that excludes a considerable portion of the population from accessing care."[119]

RELEVANT FRAMEWORKS
One Health/One Welfare

The One Health framework considers the health of people, animals, and the environment as inherently linked.[120] In 2013, the term "One Welfare" was coined to expand One Health to all aspects of human, social, and animal welfare.[121] One Welfare was then further expanded, moving beyond clinical considerations to describe all direct and indirect connections among the well-being of people, animals, and the environment.[122,123] The concept of integral connections among people, animals, and the environment has existed for millennia in Indigenous ways of knowing; in 2023, an Indigenous speaker at an animal welfare conference in Canada described One Health as "a White people way of saying Indigenous sovereignty."[124]

The One Welfare framework is useful for considering equity in practice. There are many social and environmental conditions encountered by practice teams (eg, poverty, animal hoarding, natural disasters, and houselessness) where people and animals face challenges together,[38,39,122,125,126] requiring considering broader conditions to provide animal health care. Impacts of veterinary practices extend beyond clients and patients.[4,23,127] Environmental outputs from veterinary practices that lead to environmental degradation and global warming disproportionately impact marginalized communities, and practices should consider both environmental sustainability and environmental justice.[4,23,126,127] Every organization also has a social impact; to ensure equity, practices must engage with community members, understand impacts on equity-seeking groups, and actively strive to reduce barriers.[4,7,23]

Systems of Power

Power is held by individuals and built into institutions and systems.[4] A practice that centers equity must include an awareness of power dynamics at all levels and a willingness to acknowledge, use, and share or cede power to achieve more equitable outcomes.[4] Privilege in a workplace comes from access to various forms of power, including being part of a socially advantaged group, having specific expertise, and/or occupying a higher position in an organizational hierarchy.[4,128] Human health care settings contain powerfully entrenched status hierarchies, with doctors elevated above other team members[129]; this is also reflected in veterinary health care settings.[90,130]

There is also an inherent power differential between veterinary health care teams and their clients, which has traditionally resulted in paternalistic models of care. In human medicine, a "shared decision-making (SDM)" model that integrates physician expertise with patient autonomy, improving patient outcomes, has recently gained widespread acceptance.[131] In veterinary medicine, these principles are adopted by the relationship-centered care model, which flattens the hierarchy between veterinary service providers and clients and recognizes clients as experts on their own human–animal families.[41,132] Relationship-centered care is a trusting and collaborative partnership where veterinary teams optimize outcomes using open-ended questions and reflective listening to exchange information.[132] In one survey, 74.2% of pet owners preferred an SDM-based model, whereas only 14.6% favored a paternalistic model of communication.[132] Despite rising awareness and client preference for relationship-centered care, many veterinarians still use paternalistic roles and communication styles with clients.[133,134]

The Role of Trust

Trust is important for both client interactions and workplace teams.[4,51] In human medicine, trust in providers improves patient outcomes and collaborative decision-making.[135] For veterinary teams, work culture, including a high level of trust in the employer, is important in predicting well-being and reducing burnout and psychological distress.[51] Workplaces can be high-trust, medium-trust, or low-trust environments, with trust being a direct result of how leaders have responded to incidents of harm, feedback, and challenges.[4]

Achieving equity in a workplace is easiest in high-trust environments; in a medium-trust setting, leaders will need to build trust through enhanced accountability and engagement at all levels.[4] In a low-trust setting, "the status quo of structure, culture, and strategy in the organization is fundamentally inequitable," psychological safety is lacking, and team members are cynical due to fear-based decisions and repeated breaches of trust.[4] Trust must be restored before change is possible; this involves a genuine commitment to cede power to those without formal power.[4]

The Role of Trauma

"Recently, while my coworker was restraining a difficult animal, they said, don't make me 'George Floyd' you."[53]

Veterinary team members, clients, and community members who identify with a systemically excluded group or groups are not at higher risk of various poor outcomes *because of* their identity or identities; rather, these risks come from systemic oppression, social marginalization and trauma from other people, structures, and systems that have intentionally placed people and groups with specific identities at risk. Experiences of trauma, including trust violations, are lasting and can impact future perceptions and patterns of behavior.[136] Trauma has persistent and profound impacts on cognition, behavior, relationships, and physical and mental health.[136,137]

Racial trauma is recurrent, complex, and ubiquitous for racialized people and is defined as "experiences related to threats, prejudices, harm, shame, humiliation, and guilt associated with various types of racial discrimination, either for direct victims or witnesses (**Fig. 1**)."[137] These experiences can be "everyday" occurrences such as microaggressions, or "major discrimination," that is, more blatant and impactful occurrences of discrimination in health care, education, and employment.[137,138] Health care discrimination in human medicine is often based on stereotyping and reduces seeking and obtaining care, perpetuating further cycles of poor health care outcomes[138,139]; the same is likely true in veterinary medicine.

In addition to accumulated threats of everyday and major discrimination, people who identify as part of a systemically excluded group or groups can be adversely impacted by "mega-threats." These are defined as "negative, large-scale, diversity-related episodes that receive significant media attention."[140] Examples of mega-threats include legislation targeting trans youth, mass hate crimes, and murders of Black people by police.[140,141] The negative impact of a mega-threat is greatest on people who identify strongly with targeted individuals or groups, to whom these threats send a message of danger, hostility, and rejection.[141] Team members impacted by mega-threats may shift the balance of their social identity and their organizational, or work, identity, such that their social identity becomes more "activated," which may be associated with speaking out about issues about which they would normally remain silent due to workplace norms.[140] When this occurs, both internal and external safety are lacking, and it is recommended that leaders respond with acknowledgment, compassion, and support.[140]

In addition to trauma originating from broader social issues, veterinary medical providers are exposed to other forms of trauma, for example, direct and vicarious/secondary traumatic stress (indirect, involving suffering of others or animals and an inability to manage the exposure to this pain).[142,143] A trauma-informed approach that assumes the possibility of trauma and shifts the inquiry from "What's wrong with you?" to "What happened to you?" can benefit both colleagues and clients/members of the public.[41,142]

Veterinary professionals also frequently experience moral injury and moral distress when resources do not match needs and when discussing end-of-life decisions.[0,144–147] This may be exacerbated when coupled with exposure to oppression, particularly if a practitioner shares an identity with an affected person (eg, a veterinarian mother treating a sick kitten of a single mother with limited treatment funds). Moral distress occurs when a practitioner knows how to proceed, but is unable to follow that path, whereas moral injury results from protracted experiences of moral

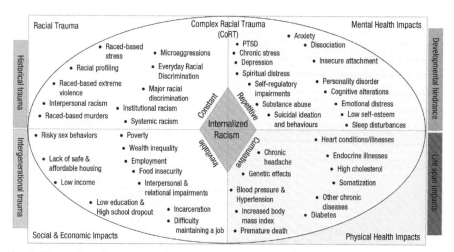

Fig. 1. Theoretical framework of complex racial trauma with examples of impacts. (*From* Cénat 2023, with permission.[137])

distress, leading to reduced mental health and functioning.[144,145] Economic euthanasia requests are a major source of burnout and moral injury; in one study, 20% of euthanasias were economic and contributed to provider burnout.[52]

SUMMARY

Understanding inequities and barriers impacting veterinary team members and the broader community is a prerequisite to building equitable practices. Veterinary team members who identify with one or more systemically excluded groups contribute valuable lived experiences, skills, and empathy but report experiencing widespread workplace discrimination and harm, perpetuated by leaders, peers, and members of the public. Due to broad socioeconomic disparities, clients and community members facing barriers to accessing care for cost or other reasons are disproportionately likely to be from systemically excluded groups. Interrogating systems of power and considering the role of trauma are necessary to move toward truly equitable solutions.

CLINICS CARE POINTS

Pearls
- Everyone in veterinary medicine, especially people with relatively privileged identities, should be aware of and understand historical and present-day inequities and the SDoH and how they impact veterinary team members, clients, and the broader community.
- The One Welfare framework considers connections between the health of people, animals, and the environment and can be used when considering the social and environmental impacts of veterinary practice.
- Systems of power and associated hierarchies influence interactions at all levels of veterinary practice, including between providers and clients, and should always be considered when using an equity lens.

Pitfalls
- Some forms of discrimination are more overt than others; intentional awareness should be applied to recognize and interrupt common "socially acceptable" forms such as accent discrimination and ageism.
- Common practice situations such as economic euthanasia can cause profound moral injury to providers, which may be compounded by the contributing role of systems of oppression.
- Veterinary practice teams may be unintentionally perpetuating inequity against members of the public through judgment, paternalistic communication, imposing preventable barriers to care, and using statements like "pet ownership is a privilege, not a right."

GLOSSARY
Definitions of Equity, Diversity, and Inclusion Terms

Terminology used in Part 1 and Part 2	
Term	Definition
2SLGBTQIA+	"This acronym stands for: Two-Spirit, Lesbian, Gay, Bisexual, Trans, Queer (or Questioning), Intersex, Asexual. The plus sign (+) represents all the different, new and growing ways that people might identify with, as well as the ways that we continually expand our understanding of sexual and gender diversity."[16] Note: this Canadian term honors "sexual and gender diversity in Indigenous cultures"[16] and "recognizes Two-Spirit people as the

(continued on next page)

Term	Definition
(continued)	
	first 2SLBTQI communities"[148] and is used in this document unless referring to a study that used different terminology
Belonging	"A fundamental human need and motivation guided by a desire to be affiliated with and respected by others that we seek to acquire and maintain throughout the life course. If inclusion is the process of creating a culture/environment that allows individuals to feel valued, then belonging is the feeling of connectedness and respect one may experience when inclusivity efforts are successful."[7,149]
Bias	"Partiality: an inclination or predisposition for or against something. Motivational and cognitive biases are 2 main categories studied in decision-making analysis. Motivational biases are conclusions drawn due to self-interest, social pressures, or organization-based needs, whereas cognitive biases are judgments that go against what is considered rational, and some of these are attributed to implicit reasoning."[150] Bias for or against an individual or group can interfere with impartial judgment.[151]
Centering (voices)	"Uplifting, trusting, and valuing the lived experiences of the people most impacted by the issue(s) and inequity(ies) you want to address; the process of centering the voices of those who have been historically marginalized."[8]
Cultural humility	"The commitment to self-evaluation and critique, to redressing the power imbalances in the provider-client dynamic, and to developing mutually beneficial and non-paternalistic partnerships with communities on behalf of individuals and defined populations."[7,8]
Deficit-based approach	Perspective that focuses on the problems of an individual or community and attempts to identify specific solutions. This unsustainable approach waits to address problems until after they have already occurred, fosters dependency on external support, and perpetuates cycles of fear, powerlessness, and poor outcomes[40,152]
Discrimination	"The differential treatment of the members of different gender, racial, ethnic, religious, national, or other groups. Discrimination is usually the behavioral manifestation of prejudice and therefore involves negative, hostile, and injurious treatment of the members of rejected groups."[150]
Diversity	"Refers to the identities we carry, including race, gender, sexual orientation, class, age, country of origin, education, religion, geography, physical or cognitive abilities, or other characteristics; valuing diversity means recognizing differences between people, acknowledging that these differences are a valued asset, and striving for diverse representation as a critical step toward equity."[7,8]
Inclusion	"A state of being valued, respected, and supported; the process of creating a culture and environment that allows individuals to feel valued for their unique qualities and experience a sense of belonging."[7,8]

(continued on next page)

(continued)	
Term	**Definition**
Intersectionality	"The complex, cumulative way in which the effects of multiple forms of discrimination (such as racism, sexism, and classism) combine, overlap, or intersect, and their multiple effects on the same individuals or groups. Also refers to the view that overlapping and interdependent systems of discrimination and inequality can more effectively be addressed together."[3,153]
One Health	"One Health is a collaborative, multisectoral, and transdisciplinary approach—working at the local, regional, national, and global levels—with the goal of achieving optimal health outcomes recognizing the interconnection between people, animals, plants, and their shared environment."[120]
One Welfare	"'One Welfare' builds on the One Health concept and is a way to recognize the many social interconnections between human welfare, animal welfare and the integrity of the environment. In practice, it is also a call for a coordinated program of action: to improve human welfare in order to improve animal welfare (and vice versa), to coordinate actions between animal welfare, human mental health, and other services, and support environmental stewardship as a fundamental step for both human and animal welfare."[123]
Performativity	"Performativity is the practice of doing equity work for compliance or to make an organization or person "look good" and increase its/their social capital vs making genuine efforts to create substantive change. Tokenism, a type of performativity, is when inclusion or diversity are pursued in a perfunctory or symbolic fashion. An example of tokenism is the recruitment of individuals from underrepresented groups to create an appearance of diversity without also taking steps to address underlying inequities."[154]
Positionality/social position	"Refers to our individual identities and the intersection of those identities and statuses with systems of privilege and oppression; shapes our psychological experiences, worldview, perceptions others have of us, social relationship, and access to resources; includes how an individual actively understands and negotiates the ways that our identities affect our relationships because of power dynamics related to privilege and oppression."[7,150]
Power	"The ability or authority to influence and make decisions that impact other people; power is often held by those who have privilege, which is a set of advantages systemically conferred on a particular person or group of people."[7,8]
Privilege	"An unearned, sustained advantage that comes from race, gender, sexuality, ability, socioeconomic status, age, and other differences."[153] These advantages and power are "derived from the historical oppression and exploitation of other groups."[3,151]
Psychological safety	The sense that people are valued, can be themselves, take risks, and raise concerns without fear of repercussions. In a culture of psychological safety, leaders intentionally foster learning and innovation, and people openly discuss mistakes, problems, and tough issues.[3,155]

(continued on next page)

(continued)

Term	Definition
Racism	A social system of advantage and oppression based on race that "penetrates every aspect of personal, cultural, and institutional life." This "includes prejudice and discrimination against, as well as exclusion, fear, suspicion, and hate of racialized people."[3]
Racialized	"Members of racialized groups are persons who do not identify as primarily white in race, ethnicity, origin, and/or color, regardless of their birthplace or citizenship. The term 'racialized' is used as a more current term than 'visible minority.' The expression recognizes that racialization is a social construct (rather than an objective biological reality)."[16]
SDoH	"Refer to the underlying community-wide social, economic, and physical conditions in which people are born, grow, live, work and age. They affect a wide range of health, functioning, and quality-of-life outcomes and risks. These determinants and their unequal distribution according to social position, result in differences in health status between population groups that are avoidable and unfair."[8]
Systemically excluded/ marginalized	"Refers to those people or groups who have been excluded or disenfranchised throughout history, and whose legacy includes day-to-day barriers that contributed to past, and perpetuate current, inequities which compound over time. Systems, policies, practices, culture, behaviors, and beliefs continue to maintain these barriers. It is often not an individual intentional, but rather a systematic, effort to discriminate. It is an unconscious, unrecognized practice of doing things as they have always been done (and recreating the historical exclusions)."[16,156]
Strengths-based approach	Perspective that focuses on the strengths and assets an individual or community has and seeks to maximize them. Rather than viewing the individual or community as the source of a problem, it recognizes contributing external factors (cultural, sociopolitical, systemic, structural, and economic). This approach creates positive cycles of empowerment, resilience, and growth.[40,152]

ACKNOWLEDGMENTS

The author is grateful to Angie Arora, Meghann Cant, Wesley Cheung, Alexandre Ellis, John Kastelic, Lexis Ly, Celeste Morales, and Jordan Woodsworth for reviewing the article prior to submission and offering suggestions that immeasurably improved the final version.

DISCLOSURE

The author has nothing to disclose.

REFLEXIVITY/POSITIONALITY STATEMENT

The author is a biracial (Chinese/White), cisgender, queer, nondisabled woman, mother, and veterinarian living with a chronic health condition. She has lived and worked in general and shelter practice in the United States and Canada. She owns a mobile and consultancy practice focused on shelter and community medicine.

REFERENCES

1. Chan A. Diversity is a fact. Equity is a choice. Inclusion is an.... Available at: https://www.linkedin.com/posts/arthurpchan_diversity-is-a-fact-equity-is-a-choice-activity-6709122719918755840-WU76. Accessed April 5, 2024.
2. Burkhard MJ, Dawkins S, Knoblaugh SE, et al. Supporting diversity, equity, inclusion, and belonging to strengthen and position the veterinary profession for service, sustainability, excellence, and impact. J Am Vet Med Assoc 2022; 260(11):1283–90.
3. American Association of Veterinary Medical Colleges. Diversity, Equity, and Inclusion Glossary. Available at: https://www.aavmc.org/wp-content/uploads/2021/08/Monograph-DEI-Glossary-01.pdf. Accessed May 1, 2024.
4. Zheng L. DEI deconstructed: your no-nonsense guide to doing the work and doing it right. Paperback edition. Oakland: Berrett-Koehler Publishers; 2024.
5. Marcano V. Creating inclusive spaces in the veterinary profession. Available at: https://veterinaryce.petdesk.com/creating-inclusive-spaces-in-the-veterinary-profession. Accessed March 27, 2024.
6. Diversity, equity and inclusion glossary. College of the Environment. Available at: https://environment.uw.edu/about/diversity-equity-inclusion/tools-and-additional-resources/glossary-dei-concepts. Accessed May 1, 2024.
7. Hawes S, Gutierrez L, Rojas L, et al. Diversity, equity, inclusion, and belonging in human-animal interactions. In: The Routledge international Handbook of human-animal interactions and Anthrozoology. New York: Taylor & Francis Group; 2024. p. 123–38.
8. Advancing health equity: a guide to language, narrative and concepts. Available at: https://www.ama-assn.org/system/files/ama-aamc-equity-guide.pdf. Accessed May 2, 2024.
9. Blackwell MJ, O'Reilly A. Access to veterinary care–a national family crisis and case for one health. Adv Small Anim Care 2023;4(1):145–57.
10. Access to veterinary care coalition report. Available at: https://pphe.utk.edu/wp-content/uploads/2020/09/avcc-report.pdf. Accessed May 1, 2024.
11. What is Health Equity? | Health Equity | CDC. 2023. Available at: https://www.cdc.gov/healthequity/whatis/index.html. Accessed April 5, 2024.
12. Marketing H. What are the Different Types of Veterinarians? Animal Care Center. 2021. Available at: https://animalcarecentersmyrna.com/what-are-the-different-types-of-veterinarians/. Accessed April 5, 2024.
13. What are the different kinds of Veterinary Jobs & Careers? :: VET&PET Jobs Marketplace. 2022. Available at: https://www.veterinaryjobsmarketplace.co.uk/blog/uk-what-are-the-different-kinds-of-veterinary-jobs-and-careers/. Accessed April 5, 2024.
14. Practice Definition & Meaning - Merriam-Webster. Available at: https://www.merriam-webster.com/dictionary/practice#:~:text=intransitiveverb,dorepeated exercisesforproficiency. Accessed April 5, 2024.
15. Fogarty CT, Mauksch LB. That's why they call it practice. Fam Syst Health 2014; 32(4):365–6.
16. Equity and inclusion glossary of terms. UBC Equity & Inclusion Office. Available at: https://equity.ubc.ca/resources/equity-inclusion-glossary-of-terms/. Accessed April 9, 2024.

17. Summers OS, Medcalf R, Hubbard KA, et al. A cross-sectional study examining perceptions of discriminatory behaviors experienced and witnessed by veterinary students undertaking clinical extra-mural studies. Front Vet Sci 2023;10. https://doi.org/10.3389/fvets.2023.940836.

18. Diversity & Inclusion on Air: Substance Abuse & Recovery. 2024. Available at: https://www.youtube.com/watch?v=IzPGFbtyc_E. Accessed May 1, 2024.

19. Racialized Minorities. Available at: https://www.thecanadianencyclopedia.ca/en/article/racialized-minorities. Accessed April 8, 2024.

20. Under Suspicion: Research and consultation report on racial profiling in Ontario. Available at: https://www.ohrc.on.ca/en/under-suspicion-research-and-consultation-report-racial-profiling-ontario/1-introduction#:~.text=%E2%80%9CRacialization%E2%80%9DistheE2%80%9Cprocess,expressesraceasasocial. Accessed April 8, 2024.

21. Government of Canada PS and PC. Guide on Equity, Diversity and Inclusion Terminology. 2024. Available at: https://www.noslangues-ourlanguages.gc.ca/en/publications/equite-diversite-inclusion-equity-diversity-inclusion-eng. Accessed April 15, 2024.

22. Race and ethnicity: evolving terminology. HillNotes. 2022. Available at: https://hillnotes.ca/2022/01/31/race-and-ethnicity-evolving-terminology/. Accessed April 9, 2024.

23. Jenkins JLJ, Rudd ML. Decolonizing animal welfare through a social justice framework. Front Vet Sci 2022;8. https://doi.org/10.3389/fvets.2021.787555.

24. Asare JZG. Decentering whiteness in the workplace: a Guide for equity and inclusion. First edition. Oakland: Berrett-Koehler Publishers; 2023.

25. U.S. Census Bureau QuickFacts. Available at: https://www.census.gov/quickfacts/fact/table/US/PST045222accessed2/8. Accessed April 9, 2024.

26. Deer K. Kanien'kohá:ka veterinarian hopes to inspire more Indigenous people into the profession. CBC News. 2022. Available at: https://www.cbc.ca/news/indigenous/indigenous-veterinarian-1.6402204. Accessed April 5, 2024.

27. Black Veterinary Association of Canada. Black Veterinary Association of Canada. Available at: https://www.bvac.ca. Accessed April 14, 2024.

28. Government of Canada SC. Visible minority and population group by generation status: Canada, provinces and territories, census metropolitan areas and census agglomerations with parts. Available at: https://www150.statcan.gc.ca/t1/tbl1/en/tv.action?pid=9810032401. Accessed April 9, 2024.

29. Government of Canada SC. Population estimates on July 1, by age and gender. 2018. Available at: https://www150.statcan.gc.ca/t1/tbl1/en/tv.action?pid=1710000501. Accessed May 2, 2024.

30. Natives in VetMed. Available at: https://www.nativesinvetmed.org. Accessed April 14, 2024.

31. Employed persons by detailed occupation, sex, race, and Hispanic or Latino ethnicity. Available at: https://www.bls.gov/cps/cpsaat11.pdf. Accessed April 9, 2024.

32. Statistics. Canadian Veterinary Medical Association. Available at: https://www.canadianveterinarians.net/about-cvma/media-centre/statistics/. Accessed April 9, 2024.

33. Brown A. About half of U.S. pet owners say their pets are as much a part of their family as a human member. Pew Research Center. Available at: https://www.pewresearch.org/short-reads/2023/07/07/about-half-us-of-pet-owners-say-their-pets-are-as-much-a-part-of-their-family-as-a-human-member/. Accessed April 9, 2024.

34. Williams DR, Priest N, Anderson NB. Understanding associations among race, socioeconomic status, and health: Patterns and prospects. Health Psychol 2016;35(4):407–11.
35. Government of Canada D of J. Cultural Diversity in Canada: The social construction of racial difference. 2003. Available at: https://www.justice.gc.ca/eng/rp-pr/csj-sjc/jsp-sjp/rp02_8-dr02_8/p6.html. Accessed April 11, 2024.
36. Barriers to Indigenous Wealth. BECU. Available at: https://www.becu.org/blog/barriers-to-indigenous-wealth. Accessed April 11, 2024.
37. Roberts C, Woodsworth J, Carlson K, et al. Defining the term "underserved:" A scoping review towards a standardized description of inadequate access to veterinary services. Can Vet J 2023;64(10):941–50.
38. Lem M. Serving homeless populations through a One Health approach. Can Vet J 2019;60(10):1119–20.
39. Card C, Epp T, Lem M. Exploring the social determinants of animal health. J Vet Med Educ 2018;45(4):437–47.
40. Shea H. Strengths v. deficit approaches to community health. Aacimotaatiiyankwi. 2021. Available at: https://aacimotaatiiyankwi.org/2021/08/10/strengths-v-deficit-approaches-to-community-health/. Accessed April 9, 2024.
41. Implementing a culturally safe & trauma-informed approach. Available at: https://traumainformed.thinkific.com/courses/implementing-a-culturally-safe-trauma-informed-approach-in-the-animal-services-sector. Accessed May 2, 2024.
42. Dhunna S, Tarasuk V. Black–white racial disparities in household food insecurity from 2005 to 2014, Canada. Can J Public Health 2021;112(5):888–902.
43. Graham S, Muir NM, Formsma JW, et al. First nations, inuit and métis peoples living in urban areas of Canada and their access to healthcare: a systematic review. Int J Environ Res Publ Health 2023;20(11):5956.
44. Howard J. Gender Pay Gap in Canada | Canadian Women's Foundation. Canadian Women's Foundation. Available at: https://canadianwomen.org/the-facts/the-gender-pay-gap/. Accessed April 15, 2024.
45. Research finds that 2SLGBTQIA+ Canadians face a wage gap. Alberta Living Wage Network. Available at: https://www.livingwagealberta.ca/news/research-finds-that-2slgbtqia-canadians-face-a-wage-gap. Accessed April 15, 2024.
46. Jajtner KM, Mitra S, Fountain C, et al. Rising income inequality through a disability lens: trends in the United States 1981–2018. Soc Indicat Res 2020;151(1):81–114.
47. Goodman N, Morris M, Boston K. Financial inequality: disability, race and poverty in America. Available at: https://www.nationaldisabilityinstitute.org/wp-content/uploads/2019/02/disability-race-poverty-in-america.pdf. Accessed April 4, 2024.
48. New Report Identifies Root Causes of Health Inequity in the U.S., Outlines Solutions for Communities to Advance Health Equity | National Academies. Available at: https://www.nationalacademies.org/news/2017/01/new-report-identifies-root-causes-of-health-inequity-in-the-us-outlines-solutions-for-communities-to-advance-health-equity. Accessed May 2, 2024.
49. Wilkerson I. Caste: the origins of our Discontents. First edition. New York: Random House; 2020.
50. Veterinary educational debt varies by sector, race | American Veterinary Medical Association. Available at: https://www.avma.org/javma-news/2021-05-15/veterinary-educational-debt-varies-sector-race. Accessed April 14, 2024.
51. Volk JO, Schimmack U, Strand EB, et al. Executive summary of the Merck Animal Health Veterinarian Wellbeing Study III and Veterinary Support Staff Study. J Am Vet Med Assoc 2022;260(12):1547–53.

52. Galaxy Vets. Veterinary burnout survey results by galaxy vets. Available at: https://galaxyvets.com/the-emotional-toll-of-financial-stress-work-environment-and-euthanasia/. Accessed April 5, 2024.

53. Multicultural Veterinary Medical Association. A profession in crisis: discrimination in veterinary medicine. 2020. Available at: https://www.youtube.com/watch?v=j7PI4YX_QNc. Accessed April 14, 2024.

54. Chung GH, Armitage-Chan E. Student experience and ethnic diversity: the experiences of underrepresented minority students at a veterinary University in the United Kingdom. J Vet Med Educ 2022;49(3):363–71.

55. Shastri T. Equity, diversity and inclusion survey results. Ont Vet Medical Assoc Mag. 2023;18–20.

56. Cheung W. Accent discrimination in the veterinary and shelter industry. Silverdale, WA: Presented at: Multicultural Veterinary Medical Association RISE Annual Conference; 2022.

57. Coupland N, Bishop H. Ideologised values for British accents1. J Sociol 2007; 11(1):74–93.

58. Accent-Bias-Britain-Report-2020.pdf. Available at: https://accentbiasbritain.org/wp-content/uploads/2020/03/Accent-Bias-Britain-Report-2020.pdf. Accessed May 2, 2024.

59. Dovchin S. The psychological damages of linguistic racism and international students in Australia. Int J Biling Educ BiLing 2020. Available at: https://www.tandfonline.com/doi/abs/10.1080/13670050.2020.1759504. Accessed May 2, 2024.

60. King E, Henning J, Green WJ, et al. Am I being understood? veterinary students' perceptions of the relationship between their language background, communication ability, and clinical learning. J Vet Med Educ 2019;46(1):35–44.

61. Singh B. Foreign-trained veterinarians and the Canadian veterinary medical establishment. Can Vet J 2007;48(9):946.

62. Whiting TL. Veterinary Practice — The Canadian multinational veterinary workforce. Can Vet J 2021;62(11):1195–201.

63. Knights D, Clarke C. Gendered practices in veterinary organisations. Vet Rec 2019;185(13):407.

64. Begeny CT, Ryan M. Gender Discrimination in the Veterinary Profession: A Brief Report of the BVA Employers' Study 2018. British Veterinary Association. 2018. Available at: https://ore.exeter.ac.uk/repository/handle/10871/36424. Accessed March 28, 2024.

65. Freestone K, Remnant J, Gummery E. Gender discrimination of veterinary students and its impact on career aspiration: A mixed methods approach. Vet Rec Open 2022;9(1):e47.

66. British Veterinary Association. Available at: https://www.bva.co.uk/media/2991/bva-report-on-discrimination-in-the-veterinary-profession.pdf. Accessed March 27, 2024.

67. Castro SM, Armitage-Chan E. Career aspiration in UK veterinary students: the influences of gender, self-esteem and year of study. Vet Rec 2016;179(16):408.

68. Tindell C, Weller R, Kinnison T. Women in veterinary leadership positions: their motivations and enablers. Vet Rec 2020;186(5):155.

69. Best CO, Perret JL, Hewson J, et al. A survey of veterinarian mental health and resilience in Ontario, Canada. Can Vet J 2020;61(2):166–72.

70. Bartram DJ, Yadegarfar G, Baldwin DS. A cross-sectional study of mental health and well-being and their associations in the UK veterinary profession. Soc Psychiatr Psychiatr Epidemiol 2009;44(12):1075–85.

71. Hatch PH, Winefield HR, Christie BA, et al. Workplace stress, mental health, and burnout of veterinarians in Australia. Aust Vet J 2011;89(11):460–8.

72. Nett RJ, Witte TK, Holzbauer SM, et al. Risk factors for suicide, attitudes toward mental illness, and practice-related stressors among US veterinarians. J Am Vet Med Assoc 2015;247(8):945–55.

73. Wogan L. Gender wage gap persists in veterinary medicine. VIN.com. 2008. Available at: https://www.vin.com/doc/?id=4235063.

74. Wayne AS, Mueller MK, Rosenbaum M. Perceptions of maternal discrimination and pregnancy/postpartum experiences among veterinary mothers. Front Vet Sci 2020;7:91.

75. Molter B, Wayne A, Mueller MK, et al. Current policies and support services for pregnant and parenting veterinary medical students and house officers at united states veterinary medical training institutions. J Vet Med Educ 2019; 46(2):145–52.

76. Rosenbaum MH, Wayne AS, Molter BL, et al. Perceptions of support and policies regarding pregnancy, parenting, and family planning during veterinary training at United States veterinary medical training institutions. J Am Vet Med Assoc 2018;253(10):1281–8.

77. Adesoye T, Mangurian C, Choo EK, et al. Perceived discrimination experienced by physician mothers and desired workplace changes: a cross-sectional survey. JAMA Intern Med 2017;177(7):1033–6.

78. Kramper S, Brydon C, Carmichael KP, Chaddock HM, Gorczyca K, Witte T. "The Damage Happens … You Just Try Not to Dwell on It": Experiences of Discrimination by Gender and Sexual Minority Veterinary Professionals and Students in the US and the UK. J Vet Med Educ 2023;50(4):482–96.

79. Greenhill L, Davis K, Lowrie P, et al. Navigating diversity and inclusion in veterinary medicine. New Dir Hum-Anim Bond; 2013.

80. Witte TK, Kramper S, Carmichael KP, et al. A survey of negative mental health outcomes, workplace and school climate, and identity disclosure for lesbian, gay, bisexual, transgender, queer, questioning, and asexual veterinary professionals and students in the United States and United Kingdom. J Am Vet Med Assoc 2020;257(4):417–31.

81. Tomasi SE, Fechter-Leggett ED, Edwards NT, et al. Suicide among veterinarians in the United States from 1979 through 2015. J Am Vet Med Assoc 2019;254(1): 104–12.

82. Previtali F, Keskinen K, Niska M, et al. Ageism in working life: a scoping review on discursive approaches. Gerontol 2022;62(2):e97–111.

83. Munir F, Randall R, Yarker J, et al. The influence of employer support on employee management of chronic health conditions at work. J Occup Rehabil 2009;19(4):333–44.

84. Peña-Guzmán DM, Reynolds JM. The harm of ableism: medical error and epistemic injustice. Kennedy Inst Ethics J 2019;29(3):205–42.

85. Emswiller BB. Age discrimination and the Age Discrimination in Employment Act. J Am Vet Med Assoc 1995;206(5):633–6.

86. Allen MW, Armstrong DJ, Riemenschneider CK, et al. Making sense of the barriers women face in the information technology work force: standpoint theory, self-disclosure, and causal maps. Sex Roles 2006;54(11):831–44.

87. Episode #196 - Fighting Ageism in Your Animal Health Career, Part 1. The VET Recruiter. Available at: https://thevetrecruiter.com/podcast/episode-196-fighting-ageism-in-your-animal-health-or-veterinary-career-part-1/. Accessed March 27, 2024.

88. Burfitt J. The golden age: mature workers in the veterinary profession. Vet Practice Magazine 2017. Available at: https://www.vetpracticemag.com.au/golden-age-mature-workers-veterinary-profession/. Accessed March 27, 2024.

89. Lindsay S, Fuentes K, Ragunathan S, et al. Ableism within health care professions: a systematic review of the experiences and impact of discrimination against health care providers with disabilities. Disabil Rehabil 2023;45(17): 2715–31.

90. Foster SM, Maples EH. Occupational Stress in Veterinary Support Staff. J Vet Med Educ 2014;41(1):102–10.

91. ABVMA Equity, Diversity & Inclusion Survey: Results and Next Steps. Available at: https://abvma.in1touch.org/document/5839/385477_8.5x11_ABVMAMembers Mag_Jan-Feb_WEB.pdf. Accessed March 27, 2024.

92. Snydor LA, Carmichael IS, Blackwell LV et al. Perceptions of Discrimination and Justice Among Employees with Disabilities. Empl Responsib Rights J 2010; 22(1):5–19.

93. Kattari SK. Ableist Microaggressions and the mental health of disabled adults. Community Ment Health J 2020;56(6):1170–9.

94. Meeks LM, Pereira-Lima K, Plegue M, et al. Disability, program access, empathy and burnout in US medical students: A national study. Med Educ 2023;57(6): 523–34.

95. Bulk LY, Easterbrook A, Roberts E, et al. 'We are not anything alike': marginalization of health professionals with disabilities. Disabil Soc 2017;32(5):615–34.

96. Sheedy K. Decoding job postings: Improving accessibility for neurodivergent job seekers. LMIC-CIMT. Available at: https://lmic-cimt.ca/decoding-job-postings-improving-accessibility-for-neurodivergent-job-seekers/. Accessed April 30, 2024.

97. MEd NRMD, MD JF. What is neurodiversity? Harvard Health. 2021. Available at: https://www.health.harvard.edu/blog/what-is-neurodiversity-202111232645. Accessed March 27, 2024.

98. Smits F, Houdmont J, Hill B, et al. Mental wellbeing and psychosocial working conditions of autistic veterinary surgeons in the UK. Vet Rec 2023;193(8):e3311.

99. Neurodiversity in Veterinary Medicine. Alberta Animal Health Source. 2022. Available at: https://www.albertaanimalhealthsource.ca/content/neurodiversity-veterinary-medicine. Accessed March 27, 2024.

100. Curiosity can lead to discovery: Embracing neurodiversity | American Veterinary Medical Association. 2024. Available at: https://www.avma.org/blog/curiosity-can-lead-discovery-embracing-neurodiversity. Accessed March 27, 2024.

101. Yankowicz S. Celebrating neurodiversity in veterinary teams. Available at: https://www.dvm360.com/view/celebrating-neurodiversity-in-veterinary-teams. Accessed March 27, 2024.

102. Sprinkle M. How Embracing Neurodiversity Strengthens Us All. Available at: https://www.linkedin.com/pulse/how-embracing-neurodiversity-strengthens-us-all-megan-sprinkle-dvm-ylb6e. Accessed March 27, 2024.

103. Hackett C, Mcclendon D. Christians remain world's largest religious group, but they are declining in Europe. Pew Research Center. Available at: https://www.pewresearch.org/short-reads/2017/04/05/christians-remain-worlds-largest-religious-group-but-they-are-declining-in-europe/. Accessed April 14, 2024.

104. Scheitle CP, Frost J, Ecklund EH. The association between religious discrimination and health: disaggregating by types of discrimination experiences, religious tradition, and forms of health. J Sci Stud Relig 2023;62(4):845–68.

105. Antisemitic Attitudes in America: Topline Findings | ADL. Available at: https://www.adl.org/resources/report/antisemitic-attitudes-america-topline-findings. Accessed April 14, 2024.

106. Allison I. CAIR: New Data Shows the End of 2023 was a 'Relentless' Wave of Bias, Community Resilience is 'Impressive' -. 2024. Available at: https://www.cair.com/press_releases/cair-new-data-shows-the-end-of-2023-was-a-relentless-wave-of-bias-community-resilience-is-impressive/. Accessed April 14, 2024.

107. Nadimpalli SB, Cleland CM, Hutchinson MK, et al. The association between discrimination and the health of Sikh Asian Indians. Health Psychol 2016;35(4): 351–5.

108. Baqai B, Azam L, Davila O, et al. Religious identity discrimination in the physician workforce: insights from two national studies of muslim clinicians in the US. J Gen Intern Med 2023;38(5):1167–74.

109. Padela AI, Azam L, Murrar S, et al. Muslim American physicians' experiences with, and views on, religious discrimination and accommodation in academic medicine. Health Serv Res 2023;58(3):733–43.

110. Jacobson LS, Janke KJ, Probyn-Smith K, et al. Barriers and lack of access to veterinary care in Canada 2022. J Shelter Med Community Anim Health 2024;3(1).

111. Bunke L, Harrison S, Angliss G, et al. Establishing a working definition for veterinary care desert. J Am Vet Med Assoc 2024;262(1):1–8.

112. Bir C, Ortez M, Olynk Widmar NJ, et al. Familiarity and use of veterinary services by us resident dog and cat owners. Animals 2020;10(3):483.

113. Thompson P, Monique C, Kim PAngela B. Understanding the experiences of elderly bereaved men and the bond with their pets. Omega J Death Dying 2023;86(4):1291–311.

114. Cant M, Gordon E. BC's housing Crisis: a Crisis for pets Too. West Coast Vet; 2023. p. 52.

115. Miller H, Ward M, Beatty JA. Population characteristics of cats adopted from an urban cat shelter and the influence of physical traits and reason for surrender on length of stay. Animals 2019;9(11):940.

116. Eagan BH, Gordon E, Protopopova A. Reasons for Guardian-Relinquishment of Dogs to Shelters: Animal and Regional Predictors in British Columbia, Canada. Front Vet Sci 2022;9. https://doi.org/10.3389/fvets.2022.857634.

117. Rah H, Choi SH. Are veterinary costs and socioeconomic status risk factors for companion animal relinquishment in the Republic of Korea? Animals 2023; 13(21):3406.

118. Ly LH, Gordon E, Protopopova A. Exploring the relationship between human social deprivation and animal surrender to shelters in British Columbia, Canada. Front Vet Sci 2021;8. https://doi.org/10.3389/fvets.2021.656597.

119. Palmer C, Sandøe P, Weary D. Ethicists' commentary on attitudes towards pet ownership among people experiencing homelessness. Letter submitted by Canadian Collective for Equity in Veterinary Medicine. Available at: https://static-curis.ku.dk/portal/files/378193921/cvj_09_2023_805.pdf. Accessed April 8, 2024.

120. One Health | CDC. 2024. Available at: https://www.cdc.gov/onehealth/index.html. Accessed April 29, 2024.

121. Colonius TJ, Earley RW. One welfare: a call to develop a broader framework of thought and action. J Am Vet Med Assoc 2013;242(3):309–10.

122. Pinillos RG, Appleby MC, Manteca X, et al. One Welfare – a platform for improving human and animal welfare. Vet Rec 2016;179(16):412–3.

123. One Welfare - Animal Health Canada. Available at: https://www.animalhealthcanada.ca/work-areas/one-welfare. Accessed April 29, 2024.

124. Gray S, Howard M. Seeing the connection: Indigenous perspectives on advocacy and animal welfare. Victoria, BC: Presented at: Humane Canada Summit for Animals; 2023.

125. Stumpf BP, Calácio B, Branco BC, et al. Animal hoarding: a systematic review. Br J Psychiatry 2023;45(4):356–65.

126. Protopopova A, Ly LH, Eagan BH, et al. Climate change and companion animals: identifying links and opportunities for mitigation and adaptation strategies. Integr Comp Biol 2021;61(1):166–81.

127. Stephen C, Carron M, Stemshorn B. Climate Change and Veterinary Medicine: Action is needed to retain social relevance. Can Vet J 2019;60(12):1356–8.

128. Pre-reading for developing an anti-oppressive practice. Available at: https://uwaterloo.ca/equity-diversity-inclusion-anti-racism/sites/default/files/uploads/documento/pro reading-for-developing-an-anti-oppressive-practice.pdf. Accessed May 2, 2024.

129. Noyes AL. Navigating the hierarchy: communicating power relationships in collaborative health care groups. Manag Commun Q 2022;36(1):62–91.

130. Kinnison T, May SA, Guile D. Inter-professional practice: from veterinarian to the veterinary team. J Vet Med Educ 2014;41(2):172–8.

131. Drolet BC, White CL. Selective paternalism. AMA J Ethics 2012;14(7):582–8.

132. Küper AM, Merle R. Being nice is not enough-exploring relationship-centered veterinary care with structural equation modeling. a quantitative study on german pet owners' perception. Front Vet Sci 2019;6. https://doi.org/10.3389/fvets.2019.00056.

133. Bard AM, Main DCJ, Haase AM, et al. The future of veterinary communication: Partnership or persuasion? A qualitative investigation of veterinary communication in the pursuit of client behaviour change. PLoS One 2017;12(3):e0171380.

134. Shaw JR, Bonnett BN, Adams CL, et al. Veterinarian-client-patient communication patterns used during clinical appointments in companion animal practice. J Am Vet Med Assoc 2006;228(5):714–21.

135. Huang ECH, Pu C, Chou YJ, et al. Public trust in physicians—health care commodification as a possible deteriorating factor: cross-sectional analysis of 23 countries. Inq J Health Care Organ Provis Financ 2018;55. 0046958018759174.

136. Van der Kolk BA. The body Keeps the Score: Brain, Mind and body in the healing of trauma. New York: Penguin Books; 2015.

137. Cénat JM. Complex Racial Trauma: Evidence, Theory, Assessment, and Treatment. Perspect Psychol Sci 2023;18(3):675–87.

138. Cénat JM, Hajizadeh S, Dalexis RD, et al. Prevalence and effects of daily and major experiences of racial discrimination and microaggressions among black individuals in Canada. 2022. Available at: https://journals.sagepub.com/doi/10.1177/08862605211023493. Accessed April 15, 2024.

139. In-Plain-Sight-Summary-Report.pdf. Available at: https://engage.gov.bc.ca/app/uploads/sites/613/2020/11/In-Plain-Sight-Summary-Report.pdf. Accessed April 15, 2024.

140. Leigh A, Melwani S. #BlackEmployeesMatter: Mega-Threats, Identity Fusion, and Enacting Positive Deviance in Organizations. Acad Manag Rev 2019;44(3):564–91.

141. Dhanani LY, Totton RR. Have you heard the news? the effects of exposure to news about recent transgender legislation on transgender youth and young adults. Sex Res Soc Pol 2023;20(4):1345–59.

142. Dolce J. It's time animal welfare adopted a trauma-informed care approach. Available at: https://www.jessicadolce.com/blog/trauma-informed-care-animal-welfare. Accessed April 15, 2024.

143. Stowman S. "Caregiver, are you alright?": The Basics of Compassion Fatigue in Veterinary Medicine. Available at: https://www.vet.upenn.edu/docs/default-source/penn-annual-conference/pac-2019-proceedings/companion-animal-track-2019/nursing-track-tue-2020/sarah-stowman—basics-of-compassion-fatigue.pdf?sfvrsn=a2f6f2ba_2. Accessed April 15, 2024.

144. Moses L, Malowney MJ, Wesley Boyd J. Ethical conflict and moral distress in veterinary practice: A survey of North American veterinarians. J Vet Intern Med 2018;32(6):2115–22.

145. Williamson V, Murphy D, Greenberg N. Experiences and impact of moral injury in U.K. veterinary professional wellbeing. Eur J Psychotraumatol 2022;13(1):2051351.

146. Williamson V, Murphy D, Greenberg N. Veterinary professionals' experiences of moral injury: A qualitative study. Vet Rec 2023;192(2):e2181.

147. Wagner B. It's Not Just Burnout: "Moral Injury" and How it Affects Veterinary Professionals. Not One More Vet. 2023. Available at: https://www.nomv.org/2023/08/19/moral-injury-and-how-it-affects-veterinary-professionals/. Accessed April 5, 2024.

148. What is 2SLGBTQI+?. 2024. Available at: https://www.canada.ca/en/women-gender-equality/free-to-be-me/what-is-2slgbtqi-plus.html. Accessed April 22, 2024.

149. Witwer RF. DEI and Belonging: Changing the Narrative and Creating a Culture of Belonging in Nonprofit Organization. Available at: https://bpb-us-w2.wpmucdn.com/usfblogs.usfca.edu/dist/9/244/files/2021/05/witwerrakiya_6199833_68188178_Rakiya-Witwer-622-Capstone-Report.pdf. Accessed May 1, 2024.

150. American Psychological Association. Equity, Diversity, and Inclusion Framework. Available at: https://www.apa.org/about/apa/equity-diversity-inclusion/framework. Accessed April 24, 2024.

151. Diversity and Inclusion Dictionary | University at Albany. Available at: https://www.albany.edu/diversity-and-inclusion/campus-educational-resources/dictionary. Accessed April 25, 2024.

152. Comparison Between Asset and Deficit Based Approaches. Available at: https://www.memphis.edu/ess/module4/page3.php. Accessed April 24, 2024.

153. DIB Glossary. Available at: https://edib.harvard.edu/files/dib/files/dib_glossary.pdf. Accessed April 22, 2024.

154. Best practices in equity, diversity and inclusion in research practice and design. Available at: https://www.sshrc-crsh.gc.ca/funding-financement/nfrf-fnfr/edi-eng.aspx. Accessed May 2, 2024.

155. American Psychological Association. What is psychological safety at work? Here's how to start creating it. Available at: https://www.apa.org/topics/healthy-workplaces/psychological-safety. Accessed April 10, 2024.

156. Glossary. York University – Decolonizing, Equity, Diversity and Inclusion Strategy. Available at: https://www.yorku.ca/dedi-strategy/glossary/. Accessed May 3, 2024.

Beginning with the End in Mind

Creating a Practice that Centers Equity-Part 2

Emilia Wong Gordon, DVM, DABVP (Shelter Medicine Practice)*

KEYWORDS

- Equity • Veterinary medicine • Access to care • Discrimination • Trauma-informed
- Psychological safety • Social determinants of health

KEY POINTS

- Equity seeks to ensure that every person and non-human animal has what they need, while acknowledging the presence of barriers arising from historical exclusion and differential access to power and resources (Part 1).
- Current controversies with implications for equity include the use of noncompete clauses, the trend of increasing corporate consolidation, and veterinary team unionization attempts.
- The most frequent barrier to access to care experienced by human-animal families is financial cost; many strategies exist to mitigate this and other barriers.
- Preventing harm is easier than responding to harm once it has occurred; practices should embrace equitable systems that support people from systemically excluded groups as a default, as these will benefit all workers.
- Creating a practice that centers equity requires intentionally and proactively fostering a culture that prevents harm, enacting policies and procedures that disrupt the status quo, and working to dismantle systems of oppression.

Continued from Part 1. Glossary of Equity, Diversity, and Inclusion [EDI] terms used can be found at the end of Part 1.

CURRENT CONTROVERSIES RELATED TO SYSTEMS OF POWER

Some of the most hotly debated current topics (**Box 1**) in the veterinary profession arise because veterinary medicine is generally a commodified form of health care, meaning it is privately funded, for-profit, and accessed based on consumer payment capability.[1]

Another controversial topic is diversity messaging by business and industry entities, which often centers business success rather than social change (**Box 2**).

Haven Veterinary Services, Vancouver, British Columbia, Canada
* PO Box 45010 Dunbar, Vancouver, British Columbia V6S 2M8, Canada.
E-mail address: egordon@havenvetservices.ca

Vet Clin Small Anim 54 (2024) 959–975
https://doi.org/10.1016/j.cvsm.2024.07.018 **vetsmall.theclinics.com**
0195-5616/24/© 2024 Elsevier Inc. All rights are reserved, including those for text and data mining, AI training, and similar technologies.

Box 1
Current issues related to employer-employee power differentials and market trends

Noncompete clauses
- Noncompete clauses are currently legal and widespread in most parts of the United States and Canada, although in April 2024 the US Federal Trade Commission announced a national ban to go into effect in late 2024.[2]
- These clauses increase prices to consumers and reduce innovation and wages, increasing wage gaps for woman and racialized employees.[3]
- They also result in longer commutes, increasing costs and reducing time for other activities; commute satisfaction is also linked to employee mental health.[4]
- Noncompete clauses may also have detrimental impacts on access to veterinary care, as other fields report reducing worker mobility and availability can reduce access to care.[5]

Corporate consolidation
- The number of practices under corporate ownership in the United States and Canada has skyrocketed, with 25% of general practices and 75% of specialty practices in the United States and greater than 20% of general practices and greater than 50% of specialty practices in Canada under corporate ownership.[6–8]
- Corporate consolidation is lucrative; veterinary consolidators can generate a 4-5x return over a few years (exceeding the anticipated 3x return for private equity firms in general).[7]
- Reported benefits include cost savings, the potential to invest in improved technology, potentially increased financial sustainability, and being able to coordinate staff and care across facilities.[6,9,10]
- Data in veterinary medicine are lacking, but in human medicine, "health care industry consolidation generally raises prices and costs of health care, but quality of health care generally does not increase accordingly."[9]
- In human medicine, consolidation reduced physician autonomy, raised concerns about health care facilities becoming "margin-driven" rather than "mission-driven," negatively impacted geographic access to care, and increased physician moral distress due to "financial" and "administrative" pressures.[10]
- Increased costs of veterinary care to the consumer have vastly exceeded inflation in the past few years.[11,12]
- Some veterinarians report feeling pressure to produce more revenue to satisfy investor expectations.[12]
- Rising costs and closure of corporate hospitals that underperform financially could negatively impact access to care, particularly in underserved areas.[8]

Unionization
- Labor unions are formed to improve working conditions, wages, and benefits.[13]
- Unionization in veterinary medicine in North America is rare and limited to non-veterinarian staff.[14]
- Staff motivations to unionize include impacts of steep price increases on clients, without a proportional increase in wages.[15]
- Employees at union practices describe benefits including improved: compensation, handling of discipline and grievances, workplace safety, and employee discounts.[11,15]
- Studies on unionization in other sectors report unions improve self-rated health, as well as improving wages and benefits for union and non-union workers and reducing overall income inequality; income is an important social determinants of health (SDoH).[13,16]
- All known veterinary unionization efforts in the United States in the past 20 years have been in response to corporate practice ownership.[17] Only 2 practices had signed union contracts in the Unites States at the time of this writing, though more practices had experienced failed staff attempts to unionize.[15]
- In Canada, there are several nonprofit veterinary facilities and at least 1 privately owned facility with unionized staff.[18–20]
- Unionization efforts are typically viewed by employers as a threat, with employers often responding strongly to prevent and suppress union organizing.[21,22]
- Despite the legal and financial risks incurred by a business that closes during union negotiations, there have been several high-profile corporate practice closures in the United States associated with staff unionization efforts.[17,22,23]

Box 2
The "business case for diversity"

- Materials focused on diversity and representation in veterinary medicine often prominently feature the "business case for diversity."[24–26]

- This is based on studies which found that greater team diversity may lead to better outcomes[27–29] and recommendations from professional management consultants.[30]

- The "business" case that diversity benefits organizational performance contrasts with the "fairness case for diversity," the idea that diversity is inherently valuable based on "fairness and social justice principles."[30]

- In a recent study of Fortune 500 companies, 98.5% (404/410) of companies that provided diversity messaging used the business case.[30] Economic arguments are regarded as "more effective and legitimate than moral arguments for selling social issues like diversity."[30]

- Despite the prevalence of the business case for diversity, there are no studies in veterinary medicine and only a few studies overall assessing the impact of this messaging, with all except one focused on the dominant majority group.[30]

- Initial studies of White Americans reported that the business case for diversity led to them displaying more anti-Black bias toward job applicants and "more negative beliefs about inclusion" overall.[30–32]

- A more recent study using the business case in a conceptual scenario and focused on systemically excluded groups found that it led to fears of stereotyping and depersonalization, as well as a reduced belief that an organization is genuinely committed to diversity.[30]

- Narratives that rely on the business case for diversity in hiring may backfire, leading to harm at an individual level and reduced organizational diversity.[30]

DISCUSSION AND RECOMMENDATIONS

"When you make space for the most marginalized, everyone above that bar benefits."[33]

A final question when considering equity in practice is: **How do we remove existing barriers?**

Equity is not just the absence of harm, but the presence of thriving and well-being.[34] Furthermore, health equity is not just the absence of poor health, but a state of access to resources to attain the "highest level of health."[35] Whether in reference to veterinary team members, clients, or patients, organizational practices should be designed with this in mind. In addition to identifying and understanding the barriers and impacts of systemic oppression, it is crucial to use a "strengths-based" (as opposed to a "deficit-based") lens.[36–38] This perspective recognizes that people and communities are resourceful and have answers to problems they face within the context of complex systems.[36–38] In contrast, a deficit lens uses a reactive focus on individual problems and proposes external interventions, creating a negative cycle of fear-driven behaviors and worsened outcomes.[36,37]

There is nothing "wrong" with people who have experienced discrimination; trauma may inform approaches but should not be used to define people. Avoid further stereotyping and "savior syndrome" approaches, whether interacting with clients, students, or colleagues.[39] What drives equitable practices is not pity or benevolence; rather, it is the belief that everyone in veterinary medicine deserves access to a professional life that meets their needs and is free of harm (**Fig. 1**), and that animal caregivers and animals deserve animal health care that does the same.

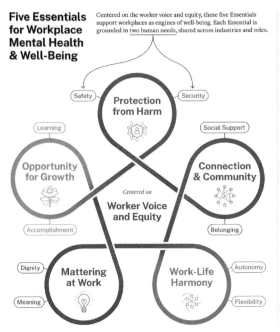

Five Essentials for Workplace Mental Health & Well-Being

Centered on the worker voice and equity, these five Essentials support workplaces as engines of well-being. Each Essential is grounded in two human needs, shared across industries and roles.

Safety — Security

Protection from Harm

Learning — Social Support

Opportunity for Growth

Connection & Community

Centered on

Worker Voice and Equity

Accomplishment — Belonging

Dignity — Autonomy

Mattering at Work   **Work-Life Harmony**

Meaning — Flexibility

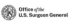 Office of the U.S. Surgeon General

Components

Creating a plan with all workers to enact these components can help reimagine workplaces as engines of well-being.

Protection from Harm
- Prioritize workplace physical and psychological safety
- Enable adequate rest
- Normalize and support mental health
- Operationalize DEIA[a] norms, policies, and programs

Connection & Community
- Create cultures of inclusion and belonging
- Cultivate trusted relationships
- Foster collaboration and teamwork

Work-Life Harmony
- Provide more autonomy over how work is done
- Make schedules as flexible and predictable as possible
- Increase access to paid leave
- Respect boundaries between work and non-work time

Mattering at Work
- Provide a living wage
- Engage workers in workplace decisions
- Build a culture of gratitude and recognition
- Connect individual work with organizational mission

Opportunity for Growth
- Offer quality training, education, and mentoring
- Foster clear, equitable pathways for career advancement
- Ensure relevant, reciprocal feedback

Fig. 1. US Surgeon General framework for workplaces, with an emphasis on protection from harm and meeting other basic human needs.[40] [a]Diversity, Equity, Inclusion and Accessibility. (*From* the Office of the U.S. Surgeon General, with permission.)

Preventing harm is easier and more effective than responding to harm after it has occurred. Studies describing the importance of employer support for workers living with disabilities and chronic illness confirm the importance of prevention; providing support after someone has experienced negative mental health impacts is less effective and the perception of "institutional betrayal" worsens outcomes.[41–44] Discrimination in veterinary medicine is vastly underreported across all systemically excluded groups, with a large majority (64%–86%) of affected people not taking action due to fear of repercussions, stigma, lack of knowledge of how to report, lack of confidence that anything would be done, and normalization of microaggressions and casual discrimination.[45–49] When a person does report, outcomes vary, but a majority of issues are not satisfactorily and definitively resolved with the affected person remaining within the organization.[46,49,50]

Though barriers and harms described above may feel daunting, huge strides in equity can be made by forming organizational culture and policies through a strengths-based lens that does not view people as the source of their problems, and centers the needs and voices of the most marginalized individuals when designing systemic solutions. The following recommendations are focused on improving workplace systems.

Veterinary Teams

> "My workplace brags about having so many employees of color, but fails to note that a vast majority of those employees are working at the lowest pay level."[51]

Formal workplace policies, organizational culture (shared behaviors and norms) and workplace climate (perception of "how it feels" to work there) are crucial to creating and maintaining equitable conditions.[52–54] All impact psychological safety, which is positively associated with mental health outcomes as well as team engagement and performance.[55,56] Both organization-led ("top-down") and employee-led ("bottom-up") elements are important to equitable organizational practices.[34,57] It may be uncomfortable to reflect on areas of privilege and disadvantage, and for leaders to share or cede power.[34,36] However, these are necessary to achieve equitable practices.

It is normal for people with relatively privileged identities to feel stressed and emotional when faced with ways that they, or people who share their identities, have caused harm in the context of systemic oppression.[36] A trauma-informed lens that considers positionality must be used during these discussions; specifically, a trauma response experienced by a person with a systemically excluded identity is "a perpetuation of harm" and should not be equated with defensive or emotional reactions of someone with a privileged identity.[36] Therefore, care should be taken to center, validate, and amplify voices of those with systemically excluded identities.[36,46,58]

Policy considerations

There are many areas where policies can promote equity, including hiring, employee management and compensation, data collection, and offboarding (**Box 3**).[34,58] Equitable hiring practices reach, engage, and offer information to a broad range of diverse candidates.[58] Workplaces with racially homogenous teams are more likely to hire candidates who are similar to hiring managers, perpetuating a lack of diversity.[34,58] Salary transparency, mandated by law in some jurisdictions, can help reduce gender and racial compensation gaps.[59,60]

Beyond considering individual needs and accommodations for specific conditions, preventive, equity-informed supports that benefit everyone and promote well-being and employee retention should be the default. When employees leave, exit interviews should be conducted and information provided should be regularly reviewed.[58,61] Feedback from people from systemically excluded groups should be actioned to drive continuous organizational improvement.[58]

Box 3
Equitable workplace policies for managers and employees

Hiring
- Include salary or reasonable range transparently in job posting.[59,60]
- Use clear, succinct language, avoid jargon, and include information about organizational culture in job postings.[62]
- Avoid gendered, racialized, or offensive language in postings.[58]
- Include only characteristics necessary to do the job; extraneous requirements may pose barriers for marginalized groups.[58]
- Do not engage in performativity or tokenism (where superficial diversity is prioritized while inequitable systems persist).[63]
- Do not use noncompete clauses.[3]
- Do not use the "business case for diversity" in messaging.[30]
- Expand recruitment beyond referral hiring.[34,58]
- Avoid discrimination based on employment gaps due to family caretaking, health, or incarceration.[58]
- Use clear criteria (ideally in a rubric) and standardized interview questions to evaluate candidates.[34,58]
- Be aware of bias, and avoid discrimination based on names and accents.[34,58]
- Include people from multiple diverse backgrounds in the interview process.[58]
- Provide training on bias, anti-racism, and anti-discrimination to employees conducting interviews.[58]
- Do not ask illegal questions (such as about family planning).[58]

Employee management.
- Provide fair compensation, including paying a living wage for the area to all employees.[40]

- Perform periodic pay audits to evaluate internal equity and ensure there are no wage gaps.[64]
- Do not prohibit, discourage, or punish discussion of compensation between employees.
- Do not suppress union organizing or take illegal action against union organizers.[22]
- Create and model boundary-setting and opportunities for rest and a healthy work-life balance.[34,46,65,66]
- Ensure role clarity and control over schedules and pace of work (recommended for neurodivergent employees, and beneficial for all employees), as well as sensory accommodations for neurodivergent employees.[67–70]
- Create collaborative written guidelines that allow autonomy for team members to make decisions, and establish clear systems (such as checklists) to prevent errors.[66]
- Provide training and support in conflict management, de-escalation, relationship-centered care, spectrum of care, trauma-informed care, cultural humility, EDI, and handling ethical dilemmas.[58,65,71,72]
- Assign tasks fairly by creating a schedule and guarding against bias; do not default to assigning women and racialized people less-glamorous tasks ("housework" vs "glamor work").[34]
- Involve team members in important decisions, and ensure diversity among participants.[73]
- Use a standardized, objective process for performance evaluations and advancement decisions, and ensure employees know how they are being evaluated.[34,58]
- Obtain performance feedback from multiple sources and include people from multiple diverse backgrounds in the evaluation process.[58]
- Provide training on bias, anti-racism, and anti-discrimination to employees conducting performance evaluations.[58]
- Conduct regular assessments of workplace culture and engagement via anonymous surveys[73] and provide opportunities for 360° feedback.[58,64]
- Avoid giving unconstructive feedback based on personality traits (women and Black/Latinx people receive less actionable and constructive feedback and more negative personality-based feedback).[64,74]
- Provide sponsorship, mentorship, and opportunities for professional development for all team members.[34,66]
- Consider how harm to employees from marginalized identities may manifest and enact safeguards to prevent harm.[58]
- Avoid dress codes and "appearance" policies (eg, restricting beards, natural hair, wearing of a head scarf, turban, or kippah, etc.) that are gendered or discriminate against racialized people and/or people who practice minority religions.[58]
- Implement time-off policies that are inclusive of various family, cultural, and religious norms; for example, parental leave that can be used for adoption, sick leave that can be used to care for an ill child or elder, floating holidays (as opposed to Christian holidays), and bereavement leave that applies to extended family (which may be needed by employees in multigenerational homes)[58] and pets.
- Offer benefits such as insurance that allow for support of dependents in multigenerational homes.
- Offer mental health days, wellness days, and mental health benefits.[34,72]
- Track outcomes to understand disparities in hiring and advancement decisions and take action.[34]
- Support team member agency and autonomy; allow schedule control and flexibility where possible, and support remote or hybrid work for positions where it is feasible.[34]
- Support employee resource groups (ERGs) and networks of team members from systemically excluded groups with resources and consideration of their needs and recommendations, and do not expect these team members to do extra unpaid work to educate others.[34,65]
- Consider diverse dietary needs, accommodate dietary restrictions, and have nonalcoholic options and spaces at work meetings and events.[33]
- Have a clear, safe, and transparent reporting and investigation process for reporting of discrimination and abuse. Ensure that reporting does not lead to negative repercussions, and commit to accountability to prevent future incidents.[46,47,73]

Offboarding
- Create a standardized offboarding checklist[61]
- Conduct exit interviews and/or surveys, review findings regularly, analyze resignation letters and other exit materials for common themes, and take action on the findings[58]
- Disaggregate results by diversity groups to understand lived experiences[58]

Culture and climate

Creating an equitable practice goes well beyond policies, as these do not always reflect how they are perceived by workers and implemented.[55] In a metareview of the effects of contextual supports for LGBT + employees, "supportive relationships" and "LGBT-supportive climate" accounted for 96% to 98% of the outcome variance in "work attitudes," "psychological strain," and "perceived discrimination" for workers, whereas formal policies explained only 2% to 4% of total variance.[55] As women, racialized people, and other systemically excluded groups are at higher risk of experiencing workplace harms that erode psychological safety, leaders must be aware of culture-related threats and act to mitigate these harms.[40,64]

Organizational culture also interacts with policies and structures and influences outcomes.[34] Culture reflects power imbalances and level of comfort with risk, feedback, mistakes, and failure.[34] Cultivating a culture of growth and feedback with a "no blame" approach can improve organizational culture and encourage reporting of mistakes.[66,75] Veterinary medical workplaces may be particularly prone to toxic cultures, where people are overworked and incivility is normalized.[66,76] Recommendations for promoting a culture that supports psychological safety are in **Box 4**.

Box 4
Recommendations to promote a culture supporting psychological safety

Proactive/preventive
- Articulate the core values of the practice, and act transparently and consistently in alignment with these values; everyone including doctors, managers, and others who hold more power in the organizational hierarchy should follow the same rules.[66,76]
- Establish and model communication expectations: communication should be clear, regular, and respectful.[66]
- Facilitate opportunities for creation and maintenance of supportive work interactions and relationships, which are highly associated with "work attitudes and well-being" for LGBT+ employees and potentially for employees who identify with other systemically excluded groups.[55]
- Show appreciation regularly and strive for far more positive interactions/feedback than negative ones.[76] The optimal ratio of positive interactions to negative interactions is approximately 5:1 in both business and personal relationships.[77]
- Nourish a culture of feedback and growth. This means feedback is normalized, constructive, kind, and occurs regularly (not just when a problem occurs or at performance reviews).[66,77]
- Common models for effective feedback (both positive and negative) include frameworks such as "describe, evaluate, suggest" or "context, behavior, impact" where a description or observation is shared, then interpreted, followed by a description of the impact and recommendations for the future.[77,78]
- Encourage professional development and advancement for every position; actively combat managerial bias, and be aware that some people may be better-connected or more likely to advocate for themselves, which can lead to disparities if managers do not regularly initiate discussions about career planning.[34]
- Ensure that staffing matches workload; encourage and model setting boundaries and asking for help when needed.[72,76]
- Consider including a Veterinary Social Worker (VSW) on the team, as an employee or contractor. A VSW can help staff debrief after traumatic cases, offer employee counseling, support training on conflict management, trauma-informed care, wellness, and compassion fatigue, de-stigmatize conversations about mental health in the workplace, and offer other employee support.[79,80]
- Consider whether company investments and/or products used in the practice are supporting social, environmental, or political harm. Be aware that for trauma-based reasons, some team members may not be comfortable with company support for military and law enforcement organizations or use of products from companies who back politicians and/or causes that harm human rights.

- Have a clear policy that considers systems of power for when the company will take positions on social issues. For example, a practice may choose to support 2SLGBTQIA + Pride month without supporting calls for "Straight Pride Month"; these are not equivalent, as the first seeks to provide necessary support to a systemically excluded group and the second is a perpetuation of injustice.

Reactive (in response to a problem)
- Address violations of communication expectations, core values, and practice policies early and consistently.[76]
- Have a clear zero-tolerance policy for discrimination,[73] including abusive behavior from clients. Ensure appropriate action is always taken in response to formal reports.
- Do not punish, conceal, or encourage hiding errors; treat them as opportunities for growth and better patient outcomes.[66]
- Model and encourage allyship and advocacy; allyship includes both "confrontation" (actively interrupting acts of discrimination) and "acknowledgment" (positive support for those with marginalized identities).[55]
- Be aware of the cumulative effects of racialized trauma (and other similar forms of trauma), including microaggressions and other "everyday" occurrences, on people from systemically excluded groups.[81] An incident that may to others seem "isolated" is not experienced as a single event, but rather as repetitive and recurrent trauma.[81] This form of complex trauma can lead to post-traumatic stress disorder (PTSD) symptoms, including hypervigilance, reliving the event(s), physical reactions to reminders of the trauma, and anger.[82]
- Consider positionality and intersectionality when an incident occurs; while it is generally important to protect those with less power in the organizational hierarchy (such as by ensuring clients are not experiencing biased treatment from staff, and that staff are not experiencing abuse from management), it is also important to consider the context, behavior, and impact. In the accent discrimination example given previously, the veterinarian's boss apologized to the client, saying "she's a younger vet, sorry if she offended you."[83] This response, which favored a client over a veterinarian who was harmed, perpetuates ageism, racism, and sexism and does not align with an equitable approach.
- Be aware of the crucial role of trust and that trust violations in the form of failure to adequately respond to incidents of discrimination and abuse will lead to feelings of institutional betrayal, reduced future reporting, and a cycle of worsened outcomes.[41–44,46]
- Be aware of mega-threats that may impact employees, and respond in a supportive way.[84]

Clients and the Public

"Believing all pets deserve access to veterinary care will help drive the creation of systems to achieve this outcome."[85]

Veterinary practitioners have crucial roles in supporting health equity for companion animals and their caregivers. The Veterinarian's Oath commits the profession to act for "the benefit of society through the protection of animal health and welfare, the prevention and relief of animal suffering…"[86] At systemic, organizational, and individual levels, we must find ways to provide care for systemically excluded people and animals. Implementing practices (**Box 5**) that support these human-animal families benefit clients and may reduce psychological distress among staff. These practices are collaborative, trust-based, and centered around beliefs that caregivers who seek veterinary care are resourceful and caring.

The most frequent barrier to care is cost; many people who cannot afford care have jobs, but lack the funds to cover veterinary costs.[85] There are many ways that practices can support these clients, including various 3rd-party payment options, partnerships with non-profits, and connecting clients to resource lists.[87–89] Another crucial strategy is for providers to gain proficiency in Spectrum of Care (SOC) or contextualized care approaches, which offer a range of evidence-based options for a particular

Box 5
Equitable practice policies and actions for clients and patients

All clients and patients
- Apply a strengths-based, trauma-informed, relationship-centered approach that recognizes clients as experts on their own families and collaborates on care plans to optimize outcomes.[38,94]
- Use respectful, gentle animal handling that minimizes fear and stress, rather than employing force.[95,96]
- Give people the option to stay with their animals for diagnostics and treatment, unless there are safety reasons this is not possible.[97,98]
- Allow clients to visit hospitalized patients regularly.
- Use inclusive language on client forms and when speaking to clients; for example, do not assume that a woman client who is married has a husband.
- Share information with clients using clear language, without jargon, at a pace that is comfortable for them.[94]
- Hire staff who speak languages common in the local community; if this is not possible, use a phone-based translation service or online translation sites. If an interpreter is used, the provider should still speak directly to the client.[99]
- Discuss anticipated costs transparently at the time of care.
- Discuss pet insurance options with clients; pet insurance has been shown to increase available funds for veterinary care[100] and reduce economic euthanasia when a crisis occurs.[101]
- Ensure all team members understand Spectrum of Care (SOC) approaches, and the difference between standard of care (a legal term that simply means the minimum care that would be provided by a "reasonably prudent" practitioner)[91] versus "gold standard care," which is a maximum standard that may not be possible for every case based on financial resources, limited availability of diagnostics/technology, or other factors.[91,102] If a team provides collaborative care that aligns with client values, expectations, and beliefs, they should not feel (or be told) that they are failing.[90]
- Consider not using the term "gold standard care," as maximal care may not be suitable for every patient, and this term has unintended consequences of inducing shame, guilt, and stress and could lead to fewer animals receiving care.[102]
- Offer a calm, clean waiting area with comfortable seating (ideally seats with arms)[99] and gender-neutral, accessible bathroom facilities.
- Consider including a VSW on the team, as an employee or contractor. A VSW can help navigate difficult financial and end-of-life decisions with clients, offer pet loss support, and help with de-escalation and other client support.[79,80]
- Advocate for public and nonprofit funding to be directed toward access to veterinary care initiatives.

Clients experiencing cost barriers
- Offer nonjudgmental, empathetic support and SOC treatment plans to clients who are not able to pay for recommended treatment plans.
- Offer freely available information about ways to manage vet bills, including flyers from nonprofits, pet insurance companies, and veterinary medical associations and information on the practice website including links to various support options.[87,89]
- Offer payment plans either through the practice, or through a 3rd-party medical care financing service (try to choose a provider with low interest rates, or ensure clients are aware of high interest rates if these are unavoidable).
- Create a clinic fund for clients to donate to fellow clients in cases with cost barriers.
- Enroll in programs like AlignCare,[103] or establish partnerships with nonprofits and/or public agencies that offer grant funding and/or referrals for care to people struggling with access to care.
- Pursue a consultation with an organization that works with veterinary clinics to increase access to care, such as Open Door Veterinary Collective.[104]
- Consider providing staff with paid time to volunteer at or donating to non-profits/non-profit events that provide access to care for severely marginalized human-animal families, such as those experiencing houselessness.

- Corporate practices and industry entities may be able to donate through existing corporate giving and partnership programs.[105–107]

Clients with disabilities
- Offer accessible parking, entry and waiting areas, and other physical spaces as well as any accommodations requested by the client.[99]
- Speak directly to the client, not to their helper if one is present.[99]
- Ask what the client needs help with, and ask permission before touching a client or their mobility device.[99]
- If the client has a service animal, ask before touching the animal. Maintain excellent preventive care, and do not separate the animal from the person unless necessary. If sedatives must be given, ensure the person has support until the animal can safely return to work.[99]
- For clients who are blind or have impaired vision, narrate who is present as well as describing physical spaces and hazards. Dispense pre-measured or pre-split medications in containers with tactile indicators.[99]
- For clients who are Deaf or hard of hearing, speak clearly and facing the client with no part of the face covered. Consider using a whiteboard, tablet, email, text messaging, and other written forms of communication to support information exchange.[99]
- For clients with mobility challenges, ask how to make their visit comfortable. If a client is in a wheelchair, do not use high counters and tables; have staff sit in a chair and do examinations on the floor where possible so the client can see.[99]
- For clients with difficulty speaking, do not assume their cognition is impaired. Do not interrupt the client or complete their sentences for them. Consider using some written communication, use reflective listening, and confirm understanding.[99]
- For clients with memory loss or dementia, ensure that all instructions are written down, create calendars and schedules for ongoing/future care, use phone and email reminders, and try to identify a family member or caregiver who can help with treatments.[99]
- Depending on the client's needs and preferences, offering mobile, in-home care (or a referral to a mobile veterinary clinic or registered veterinary technician [RVT] in-home care service) may be helpful[99]

condition to increase access to care.[90] Patients, clients, and practitioners all benefit from SOC approaches; in some cases, offering a SOC approach can create additional options when the alternatives are separation of the pet from the family through economic euthanasia or relinquishment.[91] SOC approaches are also empowering for veterinary teams, as pressure to provide "gold standard" care rather than contextualized care may lead veterinary providers to feel like they are failing if clients cannot accept recommendations.[92] Beyond financial barriers, having a diverse provider team also facilitates access to care by reducing linguistic barriers, increasing cultural competence and safety, offering enhanced creative problem-solving, and fostering empathy.[43,47,93]

SUMMARY

It is particularly crucial to center equity in veterinary medicine because the field lacks multiple types of diversity and is an essential form of health care with a commodified delivery model. There are many learnings from human health care and the social sciences that can be applied in veterinary medicine to design and implement equitable practices, improve workplace culture, and facilitate access to care. A genuine commitment to equity involves acknowledgment of systems of power and historical and existing inequities, centering the voices and needs of people who have been systemically excluded, and working collectively to dismantle systems of oppression. This will enable every person in the profession to thrive, and every animal and their caregiver to access care that meets their needs.

CLINICS CARE POINTS

Pearls
- Veterinary professionals should commit to continual learning and action regarding equity-related issues and barriers, both in society, and within the profession.
- Ways to build equity into practice include articulating and upholding core values, fostering psychological safety, implementing equitable policies, and cultivating supportive relationships and workplace culture.
- Providers can reduce care disparities and improve patient outcomes by being aware of the SDoH, adopting relationship-centered and trauma-informed practices, and applying SOC approaches.

Pitfalls
- Systems of oppression are enduring and constantly reinforced; to counter this default, the needs and voices of people with systemically excluded identities should always be centered in equity discussions.
- Business "norms" such as using the business case for diversity in hiring, requiring noncompete clauses, not disclosing salary ranges in job postings, and suppressing union organizing contravene the principles of equity.
- Leaders should be mindful that failure to implement equitable practices will lead to harm, and failure to respond to harm in a consistent and accountable way will lead to cumulative trauma, feelings of institutional betrayal, and erosion of trust.

ACKNOWLEDGMENTS

The author is grateful to Angie Arora, Meghann Cant, Wesley Cheung, Alexandre Ellis, John Kastelic, Lexis Ly, Celeste Morales, and Jordan Woodsworth for reviewing the article prior to submission and offering suggestions that immeasurably improved the final version.

DISCLOSURE

The author has nothing to disclose. Reflexivity/positionality statement: The author is a biracial (Chinese/White), cisgender, queer, non-disabled woman, mother, and veterinarian living with a chronic health condition. She has lived and worked in general and shelter practice in the United States and Canada. She owns a mobile and consultancy practice focused on shelter and community medicine.

REFERENCES

1. Huang ECH, Pu C, Chou YJ, et al. Public trust in physicians—health care commodification as a possible deteriorating factor: cross-sectional analysis of 23 countries. Inq J Health Care Organ Provis Financ 2018;55. https://doi.org/10.1177/0046958018759174. 0046958018759174.
2. FTC Announces Rule Banning Noncompetes. Federal Trade Commission. 2024. Available at: https://www.ftc.gov/news-events/news/press-releases/2024/04/ftc-announces-rule-banning-noncompetes. Accessed May 2, 2024.
3. Non-Compete Clause Rule. Fed Regist. 2023. Available at: https://www.federalregister.gov/documents/2023/01/19/2023-00414/non-compete-clause-rule. Accessed April 14, 2024.
4. Olsson LE, Gärling T, Ettema D, et al. Happiness and satisfaction with work commute. Soc Indicat Res 2013;111(1):255–63.
5. Brown KJ, Brodhead MT. Reported effects of noncompete clauses on practitioners in applied behavior analysis. Behav Analyst Pract 2023;16(1):251–64.

6. Osborne D. The corporatization of veterinary medicine. Can Vet J 2023;64(5): 483–8.
7. Zak I. How veterinary consolidators are building a future-proof enterprise. Entrepreneur; 2021. Available at: https://www.entrepreneur.com/growing-a-business/how-veterinary-consolidators-are-building-a-future-proof/362267. Accessed April 15, 2024.
8. Kelly R. Pandemic hastens ongoing trend in veterinary consolidation. VIN.com; 2021. Available at: https://www.vin.com/doc/?id=4235063.
9. O'Hanlon CE. Impacts of health care industry consolidation in pittsburgh, pennsylvania: a qualitative study. Inq J Health Care Organ Provis Financ 2020;57. https://doi.org/10.1177/0046958020976246. 0046958020976246.
10. Cutler DM, Scott Morton F. Hospitals, market share, and consolidation. JAMA 2013;310(18):1964–70.
11. Nolen S. The corporatization of veterinary medicine | American Veterinary Medical Association. 2018. Available at: https://www.avma.org/javma-news/2018-12-01/corporatization-veterinary-medicine. Accessed April 15, 2024.
12. Carroll L. The high cost of corporate ownership of veterinary practices | observer. Available at: https://observer.com/2023/03/veterinary-practices-are-increasingly-corporately-owned-and-pets-owners-pay-the-price/. Accessed April 15, 2024.
13. Malinowski B, Minkler M, Stock L. Labor unions: a public health institution. Am J Publ Health 2015;105(2):261–71.
14. National Veterinary Professionals Union. NVPU. Available at: https://www.natvpu.org/. Accessed April 15, 2024.
15. Singler E. Animal hospital employee union ratifies its first contract. 2024. Available at: https://www.aaha.org/publications/newstat/articles/2024-1/animal-hospital-employee-union-ratifies-its-first-contract/. Accessed March 27, 2024.
16. Farber HS, Herbst D, Kuziemko I, et al. Unions and inequality over the twentieth century: new evidence from survey data. Q J Econ 2021;136(3):1325–85.
17. Wogan L. A sixth veterinary hospital in US votes to unionize. VIN.com; 2022. Available at: https://www.vin.com/doc/?id=4235063.
18. Gawthrop D. CUPE 1622 workers ratify new contract with BC SPCA. CUPE BC. 2023. Available at: https://www.cupe.bc.ca/2023/12/01/cupe-1622-workers-ratify-new-contract-with-bc-spca/. Accessed April 14, 2024.
19. CUPE 503 - Ottawa Humane Society. Canadian union of public employees. Available at: https://cupe.ca/local/cupe-503-ottawa-humane-society. Accessed April 14, 2024.
20. Veterinary workers join the union — UFCW 175. UFCW Canada - Canada's Private Sector Union. Available at: http://www.ufcw.ca/index.php?option=com_content&view=article&id=30181:veterinary-workers-join-the-union-ufcw-175&catid=9538&Itemid=6&lang=en. Accessed April 14, 2024.
21. Bruner R. Why American companies fight unions. TIME; 2022. Available at: https://time.com/6168898/why-companies-fight-unions/. Accessed April 14, 2024.
22. Bahat RE, Kochan T. How businesses should (and shouldn't) respond to union organizing. 2023. Available at: https://hbr.org/2023/01/how-businesses-should-and-shouldnt-respond-to-union-organizing. Accessed April 14, 2024.
23. Wogan L. Thrive to close veterinary ER hospital amid union talks - News - VIN. 2023. Available at: https://news.vin.com/default.aspx?pid=210&Id=11633319&f5=1. Accessed March 27, 2024.

24. Marcano V. Creating inclusive spaces in the veterinary profession. Available at: https://veterinaryce.petdesk.com/creating-inclusive-spaces-in-the-veterinary-profession. Accessed March 27, 2024.
25. Veterinary Medicine DEIB Resources & Articles. DVMC. Diversify Veterinary Medicine Coalition. Available at: https://diversifyvetmed.org/knowledge-center/. Accessed March 27, 2024.
26. Why diversity is good for business | American Veterinary Medical Association. Available at: https://www.avma.org/resources-tools/diversity-and-inclusion-veterinary-medicine/why-diversity-good-business. Accessed March 27, 2024.
27. Yang Y, Tian TY, Woodruff TK, et al. Gender-diverse teams produce more novel and higher-impact scientific ideas. Proc Natl Acad Sci USA 2022;119(36). e2200841119.
28. Gomez LE, Bernet P. Diversity improves performance and outcomes. J Natl Med Assoc 2019;111(4).303–92.
29. Tshetshema CT, Chan KY. A systematic literature review of the relationship between demographic diversity and innovation performance at team-level. Technol Anal Strateg Manag 2020;32(8):955–67.
30. Georgeac OAM, Rattan A. The business case for diversity backfires: Detrimental effects of organizations' instrumental diversity rhetoric for underrepresented group members' sense of belonging. J Pers Soc Psychol 2023;124(1):69–108.
31. Williams JB. Breaking down bias: Legal mandates vs. corporate interests. Wash L. Rev 2017;92:1473.
32. Trawalter S, Driskell S, Davidson MN. What is good isn't always fair: on the unintended effects of framing diversity as good. Anal Soc Issues Public Policy 2016;16(1):69–99.
33. Diversity & Inclusion on Air. Substance abuse & recovery. 2024. Available at: https://www.youtube.com/watch?v=IzPGFbtyc_E. Accessed May 1, 2024.
34. Zheng L. DEI deconstructed: your No-nonsense guide to doing the work and doing it right. Paperback edition. Oakland: Berrett-Koehler Publishers; 2024.
35. What is Health Equity?. Health equity. CDC; 2023. Available at: https://www.cdc.gov/healthequity/whatis/index.html. Accessed April 5, 2024.
36. Hawes S, Gutierrez L, Rojas L, et al. Diversity, equity, inclusion, and belonging in human-animal interactions. In: The routledge international handbook of human-animal interactions and anthrozoology. New York: Taylor & Francis Group; 2024. p. 123–38.
37. Shea H. Strengths v. deficit approaches to community health. aacimotaatiiyankwi. 2021. Available at: https://aacimotaatiiyankwi.org/2021/08/10/strengths-v-deficit-approaches-to-community-health/. Accessed April 9, 2024.
38. Implementing a culturally safe & trauma-informed approach. Available at: https://traumainformed.thinkific.com/courses/implementing-a-culturally-safe-trauma-informed-approach-in-the-animal-services-sector. Accessed May 2, 2024.
39. Gomez VM. White saviorism in veterinary medicine and how to avoid it. Available at: https://cvma.net/wp-content/uploads/2023/01/Unity_JanFeb23.pdf. Accessed May 2, 2024.
40. Workplace Mental Health & Well-Being. Current priorities of the U.S. Surgeon General. Available at: https://www.hhs.gov/surgeongeneral/priorities/workplace-well-being/index.html. Accessed May 2, 2024.
41. Lindsay S, Fuentes K, Ragunathan S, et al. Ableism within health care professions: a systematic review of the experiences and impact of discrimination

against health care providers with disabilities. Disabil Rehabil 2023;45(17): 2715–31.

42. Snyder LA, Carmichael JS, Blackwell LV, et al. Perceptions of discrimination and justice among employees with disabilities. Empl Responsib Rights J 2010; 22(1):5–19.

43. Meeks LM, Pereira-Lima K, Plegue M, et al. Disability, program access, empathy and burnout in US medical students: a national study. Med Educ 2023;57(6): 523–34.

44. Lett K, Tamaian A, Klest B. Impact of ableist microaggressions on university students with self-identified disabilities. Disabil Soc 2020;35(9):1441–56.

45. Burkhard MJ, Dawkins S, Knoblaugh SE, et al. Supporting diversity, equity, inclusion, and belonging to strengthen and position the veterinary profession for service, sustainability, excellence, and impact. J Am Vet Med Assoc 2022; 260(11):1283–90.

46. Summers OS, Medcalf R, Hubbard KA, et al. A cross-sectional study examining perceptions of discriminatory behaviors experienced and witnessed by veterinary students undertaking clinical extra-mural studies. Front Vet Sci 2023;10. https://doi.org/10.3389/fvets.2023.940836.

47. Chung GH, Armitage-Chan E. Student experience and ethnic diversity: the experiences of underrepresented minority students at a Veterinary University in the United Kingdom. J Vet Med Educ 2022;49(3):363–71.

48. Freestone K, Remnant J, Gummery E. Gender discrimination of veterinary students and its impact on career aspiration: A mixed methods approach. Vet Rec Open 2022;9(1):e47.

49. Kramper S, Brydon C, Carmichael KP, et al. "The damage happens…you just try not to dwell on it": experiences of discrimination by gender and sexual minority veterinary professionals and students in the US and the UK. J Vet Med Educ 2023;50(4):482–96.

50. British Veterinary Association. Available at: https://www.bva.co.uk/media/2991/bva-report-on-discrimination-in-the-veterinary-profession.pdf. Accessed March 27, 2024.

51. Multicultural Veterinary Medical Association. A profession in crisis: discrimination in veterinary medicine. 2020. Available at: https://www.youtube.com/watch?v=j7Pl4YX_QNc. Accessed April 14, 2024.

52. McKay PF, Avery DR, Morris MA. A tale of two climates: diversity climate from subordinates and managers perspectives and their role in store unit sales performance. Person Psychol 2009;62(4):767–91.

53. Glisson C. The role of organizational culture and climate in innovation and effectiveness. Hum Serv Organ Manag Leadersh Gov 2015;39(4):245–50.

54. Dimension: Organizational culture and climate - center for states - child welfare capacity building collaborative. Available at: https://capacity.childwelfare.gov/states/topics/cqi/organizational-capacity-guide/organizational-culture-and-climate. Accessed April 10, 2024.

55. Fletcher L, Everly BA. Perceived lesbian, gay, bisexual, and transgender (LGBT) supportive practices and the life satisfaction of LGBT employees: The roles of disclosure, authenticity at work, and identity centrality. J Occup Organ Psychol 2021 Sep;94(3):485–508. Available at: https://bpspsychub.onlinelibrary.wiley.com/doi/10.1111/joop.12336.

56. American Psychological Association. What is psychological safety at work? Here's how to start creating it. Available at: https://www.apa.org/topics/healthy-workplaces/psychological-safety. Accessed April 10, 2024.

57. Witte TK, Kramper S, Carmichael KP, et al. A survey of negative mental health outcomes, workplace and school climate, and identity disclosure for lesbian, gay, bisexual, transgender, queer, questioning, and asexual veterinary professionals and students in the United States and United Kingdom. J Am Vet Med Assoc 2020;257(4):417–31.
58. Asare JZG. Decentering whiteness in the workplace: a guide for equity and inclusion. 1st edition. Oakland: Berrett-Koehler Publishers; 2023.
59. How pay transparency can help close wage gaps in the workplace. World Economic Forum; 2023. Available at: https://www.weforum.org/agenda/2023/04/how-pay-transparency-help-close-wage-gaps-in-workplace/. Accessed April 14, 2024.
60. Baker M, Halberstam Y, Kroft K, et al. Pay transparency and the gender gap. Am Econ J Appl Econ 2023;15(2):157–83.
61. Offboarding. Definition & best practices (2024 Guide)   Forbes advisor. Available at: https://www.forbes.com/advisor/business/offboarding/. Accessed April 11, 2024.
62. Sheedy K. Decoding job postings: improving accessibility for neurodivergent job seekers. LMIC-CIMT. Available at: https://lmic-cimt.ca/decoding-job-postings-improving-accessibility-for-neurodivergent-job-seekers/. Accessed April 30, 2024.
63. Best practices in equity, diversity and inclusion in research practice and design. Available at: https://www.sshrc-crsh.gc.ca/funding-financement/nfrf-fnfr/edi-eng.aspx. Accessed May 2, 2024.
64. Agbanobi A, Asmelash TV. Creating psychological safety for black women at your company. Harv Bus Rev 2023. Available at: https://hbr.org/2023/05/creating-psychological-safety-for-black-women-at-your-company. Accessed April 12, 2024.
65. Timmenga FSL, Jansen W, Turner PV, et al. Mental well-being and diversity, equity, and inclusiveness in the veterinary profession: pathways to a more resilient profession. Front Vet Sci 2022;9. https://doi.org/10.3389/fvets.2022.888189.
66. Jurney C. How to conquer 4 toxic team cultures in veterinary practice. equimanagement. 2024. Available at: https://equimanagement.com/business-development/office-management/how-to-conquer-4-toxic-team-cultures-in-veterinary-practice/. Accessed April 11, 2024.
67. Neurodiversity in Veterinary Medicine. Alberta animal health source. 2022. Available at: https://www.albertaanimalhealthsource.ca/content/neurodiversity-veterinary-medicine. Accessed March 27, 2024.
68. Curiosity can lead to discovery: embracing neurodiversity | American Veterinary Medical Association. 2024. Available at: https://www.avma.org/blog/curiosity-can-lead-discovery-embracing-neurodiversity. Accessed March 27, 2024.
69. Yankowicz S. Celebrating neurodiversity in veterinary teams. Available at: https://www.dvm360.com/view/celebrating-neurodiversity-in-veterinary-teams. Accessed March 27, 2024.
70. Sprinkle M. How embracing neurodiversity strengthens us all. Available at: https://www.linkedin.com/pulse/how-embracing-neurodiversity-strengthens-us-all-megan-sprinkle-dvm-ylb6e. Accessed March 27, 2024.
71. Moses L, Malowney MJ, Wesley Boyd J. Ethical conflict and moral distress in veterinary practice: A survey of North American veterinarians. J Vet Intern Med 2018;32(6):2115–22.
72. Stevenson R, Morales C. Trauma in animal protection and welfare work: the potential of trauma-informed practice. Animals 2022;12(7):852.

73. Flietner MB. Stopping the pain of prejudice: the veterinary profession needs to heal itself of biased behaviors. Available at: https://www.aaha.org/publications/trends-magazine/trends-articles/2021/july-2021/stopping-the-pain-of-prejudice/. Accessed April 30, 2024.

74. Language bias in performance feedback: 2022 Data analysis and survey results. Textio. Available at: https://explore.textio.com/feedback-bias. Accessed April 12, 2024.

75. Neuspiel DR, Stubbs EH, Liggin L. Improving reporting of outpatient pediatric medical errors. Pediatrics 2011;128(6):e1608–13.

76. Moore IC, Coe JB, Adams CL, et al. Exploring the impact of toxic attitudes and a toxic environment on the veterinary healthcare team. Front Vet Sci 2015;2:78.

77. MCC DJMR. Council post: optimizing positive feedback. forbes. Available at: https://www.forbes.com/sites/forbescoachescouncil/2023/09/13/optimizing-positive-feedback/. Accessed April 18, 2024.

78. Feedback and Improvement. Becoming a better writer by helping other writers. eli review. Available at: http://elireview.com/content/students/feedback/. Accessed May 2, 2024.

79. Career spotlight: veterinary social workers | HumanePro by The Humane Society of the United States. Available at: https://humanepro.org/magazine/articles/career-spotlight-veterinary-social-workers. Accessed May 2, 2024.

80. Hoy-Gerlach J, Ojha M, Arkow P. Social workers in animal shelters: a strategy toward reducing occupational stress among animal shelter workers. Front Vet Sci 2021;8. https://doi.org/10.3389/fvets.2021.734396.

81. Cénat JM. Complex racial trauma: evidence, theory, assessment, and treatment. Perspect Psychol Sci 2023;18(3):675–87.

82. Weathers L, Huska & Keane. PCL-C for DSM-IV (11/1/94). National Center for PTSD - behavioral science division. Available at: https://www.ptsd.va.gov/professional/assessment/documents/APCLC.pdf. Accessed April 18, 2024.

83. Cheung W. Accent discrimination in the veterinary and shelter industry. Presented at: multicultural veterinary medical association annual conference; 2022.

84. Leigh A, Melwani S. #BlackEmployeesMatter: mega-threats, identity fusion, and enacting positive deviance in organizations. Acad Manag Rev 2019;44(3):564–91.

85. Blackwell MJ, O'Reilly A. Access to veterinary care–a national family crisis and case for one health. Adv Small Anim Care 2023;4(1):145–57.

86. Veterinarian's oath | American Veterinary Medical Association. Available at: https://www.avma.org/resources-tools/avma-policies/veterinarians-oath. Accessed April 12, 2024.

87. Pet help finder. Available at: https://www.pethelpfinder.org/m/phf. Accessed April 14, 2024.

88. Carlson J. Strategies to help clients pay for veterinary care. DVM 2018;360. Available at: https://www.dvm360.com/view/strategies-help-clients-pay-veterinary-care. Accessed April 14, 2024.

89. Having trouble affording your pet?. The humane society of the United States. Available at: https://www.humanesociety.org/resources/are-you-having-trouble-affording-your-pet. Accessed April 14, 2024.

90. The spectrum of care initiative. AAVMC. Available at: https://www.aavmc.org/the-spectrum-of-care-initiative/. Accessed April 15, 2024.

91. Brown CR, Garrett LD, Gilles WK, et al. Spectrum of care: more than treatment options. J Am Vet Med Assoc 2021;259(7):712–7.

92. Williamson V, Murphy D, Greenberg N. Experiences and impact of moral injury in U.K. veterinary professional wellbeing. Eur J Psychotraumatol 2022;13(1): 2051351.
93. Smits F, Houdmont J, Hill B, et al. Mental wellbeing and psychosocial working conditions of autistic veterinary surgeons in the UK. Vet Rec 2023;193(8):e3311.
94. Küper AM, Merle R. Being nice is not enough-exploring relationship-centered veterinary care with structural equation modeling. a quantitative study on german pet owners' perception. Front Vet Sci 2019;6. https://doi.org/10.3389/fvets.2019.00056.
95. Why and what is low stress handling®. CattleDog Publishing. Available at: https://cattlcdogpublishing.com/why-and-what-is-low-stress-handling/. Accessed May 3, 2024.
96. Fear free pets. Available at: https://fearfreepets.com/. Accessed May 3, 2024.
97. Davis J. Don't leave me. why, when, and how to "take pets to the back." Fear Free Pets 2019. Available at: https://fearfreepets.com/dont-leave-take-pets-back/. Accessed May 3, 2024.
98. Thornton K. Dogs less stressed with owners present at exams, study shows. fear free pets. 2021. Available at: https://fearfreepets.com/dogs-less-stressed-with-owners-present-at-exams/. Accessed May 3, 2024.
99. Grigg EK, Hart LA. Enhancing success of veterinary visits for clients with disabilities and an assistance dog or companion animal: a review. Front Vet Sci 2019;6. https://doi.org/10.3389/fvets.2019.00044.
100. Williams A, Williams B, Hansen CR, et al. The impact of pet health insurance on dog owners' spending for veterinary services. Animals 2020;10(7):1162.
101. Boller M, Nemanic TS, Anthonisz JD, et al. The effect of pet insurance on pre-surgical euthanasia of dogs with gastric dilatation-volvulus: a novel approach to quantifying economic euthanasia in veterinary emergency medicine. Front Vet Sci 2020;7. https://doi.org/10.3389/fvets.2020.590615
102. Skipper A, Gray C, Serlin R, et al. 'Gold standard care' is an unhelpful term. Vet Rec 2021;189(8):331.
103. Improving access to veterinary care. Available at: https://aligncare.com/landing. Accessed May 3, 2024.
104. Open door veterinary collective. Available at: https://opendoorconsults.org/. Accessed April 28, 2024.
105. VCA charities | supporting programs and organizations that help pets in need. Available at: https://vcacharities.org/. Accessed April 28, 2024.
106. Community support, sponsorships & corporate giving | Purina® Canada. Available at: https://www.purina.ca/about-purina/supporting-communities. Accessed April 28, 2024.
107. Zoetis foundation. Zoetis. Available at: https://www.zoetis.com/our-company/zoetis-foundation/. Accessed April 28, 2024.

Diversifying the Veterinary Technician Specialist (VTS) Pipeline

Stephen Niño Cital, RVT, SRA, RLAT, CVPP, VTS-LAM[a,b,*],
Camia Tonge, MS, LVT, VTS (SAIM)[c]

KEYWORDS

- Veterinary technician specialists - Diversity, equity, inclusion, and belonging
- Career advancement - Mentorship - Active recruitment

KEY POINTS

- Pathways and even awareness about specialization may present additional challenges for underrepresented groups.
- Awareness and discussion of the challenges we face as a profession, including those faced by Black, Indigenous, and other People of Color and other underrepresented groups, can help to impart knowledge, allyship, and cultural competency to help diversify the veterinary technician specialist (VTS) pipeline.
- Incorporating diversity, equity, inclusion and belonging as a part of long-term goals and strategic planning is needed.
- Discrimination or negative bias among those who do not pass as White is 2.4x higher than the overall discrimination or negative bias experienced by all respondents.
- Sexism (against women), ageism, racism/colorism, and body shaming were the top reasons given for discrimination.
- VTS demographics align with broader veterinary industry demographic studies showing poor diversity in the veterinary industry.

INTRODUCTION

The veterinary industry faces diversity challenges across all roles, from customer service representatives to clinical staff, to executive levels. Specific demographic studies for all of the roles within veterinary medicine are lacking with the most data available being specific to veterinarians, followed by "veterinary technicians".[1] The demographic data for veterinary technicians represented are questionable in many of the

[a] Department of Neurobiology, HHMI at Stanford University, 299 Campus Drive, Stanford, CA 94305, USA; [b] Remedy Veterinary Specialists, San Francisco, CA, USA; [c] Schwarzman Animal Medical Center, New York, NY, USA
* Corresponding author. Academy of Laboratory Animal Veterinary Technicians and Nurses.
E-mail address: matacital@gmail.com

Vet Clin Small Anim 54 (2024) 977–993
https://doi.org/10.1016/j.cvsm.2024.07.019
vetsmall.theclinics.com
0195-5616/24/© 2024 Elsevier Inc. All rights are reserved, including those for text and data mining, AI training, and similar technologies.

data sets by the lack of distinction in the surveys or analysis to delineate if the "veterinary technician" respondent is a credentialed veterinary technician (CrVT), compared to a veterinary assistant (VA).[2,3] Diversity among specialists whether, that is a veterinarian or veterinary technician specialist (VTS) is even more deficient, essentially nonexistent for those that have earned the VTS credential.

Predictions indicate that people of color will become the majority in the United States (US) by 2042.[4] Clients and veterinary professionals alike deserve representation that mirrors the growing diversity of society, which is crucial for several reasons. Firstly, it promotes a more inclusive and equitable environment where individuals from various backgrounds feel valued, empowered, and belong. This diversity cultivates innovation, creativity, and a broader range of perspectives, which are essential for addressing complex challenges in veterinary care, as well as mental well-being of staff.

Secondly, diversity enhances the quality of care provided to animals. Different cultures and communities may have unique perspectives on animal health practices. Having a diverse workforce allows for better communication and understanding of these perspectives, known as cultural competency. This, in turn, leads to more effective treatment plans and improved outcomes for patients in addition to client satisfaction.

Furthermore, diversity in veterinary medicine reflects the broader societal values of inclusivity and equity. By actively promoting diversity, equity, inclusion and belonging (DEIB), the veterinary industry can one day correct its long-standing title of being one of the least diverse professions, and may one day set an example for other professions and contribute to the overall goal of building a more just and equitable society. Like other articles within this series, this section will focus on Black, Indigenous, and other People of Color (BIPOC).[5,6]

* A note on "belonging": Belonging is based on sincere inclusion and acceptance of individuals for who they are. "Fitting in" is the opposite of belonging, which requires someone to assimilate or conform to a majority group.

WHAT IS A VETERINARY TECHNICIAN SPECIALIST?

Here we present the first ever demographic data looking at race, gender, sexual orientation, gender presentation, audible or visible characteristics, and disabilities for CrVT's that have undergone the VTS certification. But first, we must address an even bigger problem both in the veterinary industry and the general public—familiarity with what a CrVT is and appropriate utilization. With almost half (47%) of US respondents not knowing what a CrVT is, and an alarming 74% not understanding what CrVTs do on a day to day basis illustrates this.[7]

*For appropriate utilization, please refer to the first comprehensive set of guidelines for CrVT's published by the American Animal Hospital Association (AAHA) in 2023: https://www.aaha.org/aaha-guidelines/2023-aaha-technician-utilization-guidelines/home/

All too often anyone working with an animal and providing care within a veterinary premise is termed a "veterinary technician". This is incorrect. A veterinary technician is someone who is credentialed as such through a licensing, certifying, or registration process. A person who has not done the credentialing but functions similarly to a veterinary technician is known as a VA.[8] Certain states and the National Association of Veterinary Technicians in America offer certifications for VAs. Some veterinary practices may even consider entry-level care staff as "technician assistants." As described earlier, it is still common for many members of the public to not understand what a CrVT is, let alone the steps needed to pursue this career path. Educating children and young adults about this career path is largely lacking or focuses on becoming a veterinarian. In fact, many of the affinity groups for BIPOC veterinary professionals still only focus on promoting veterinary medicine from the veterinarian's perspective. Once the public and the veterinary profession itself better understands all the various roles in veterinary medicine we can have a more thoughtful conversation on increasing diversity among the different roles available in the veterinary industry.

Currently, there are 16 approved veterinary technician specialty academies. These specialty academies are recognized by the American Veterinary Medical Association (AVMA) and National Association for Veterinary Technicians in America (NAVTA). NAVTA's committee on veterinary technician specialties (CVTS) oversees and regulates standardized policies all VTS academies must abide by to maintain recognition. This was modeled after the American Board of Veterinary Specialties' approval and recognition process.[9]

Each specialty academy has slightly different requirements but at minimum requires an applicant to have passed the national or a state's veterinary technician examination and maintain their credential in good standing. This commonly requires graduation from a 2^2 or 4^4 y AVMA-accredited veterinary technology program. The road to becoming a VTS also requires no less than 3 to 5 y of practical clinical experience at an advanced level. After a minimum number of years of work with a majority (>70%) of that time focused on the specialty of interest, and under the supervision of a licensed veterinarian—who is often a board-certified veterinary specialist—an interested CrVT may start the application process. There are currently 28 specialties offered from the 16 approved academies.

*Information on the specialties offered can be found here: https://navta.net/veterinary-technician-specialties/

The VTS application process includes demonstrating to the specialty academy's credentialing committee that the applicant has worked a majority of their time in the area of specialization in the 3 to 5 y preceding their application date. Applicants then have a 1-year period to log a minimum of 50 or more cases where they demonstrate mastery of the academy's required skills. Academies mandate documentation of the applicants' case work throughout their application year, along with a veterinarian or VTS attestation that the skills demonstrated have been mastered. Applicants must also submit case reports colected from the log or census of cases seen during the application year. These reports must be written at a professional, publication-ready level, providing details of case management, and highlighting the applicants' advanced knowledge, critical thinking skills, and how the application of their mastered skills and knowledge impacted the course of the patient's treatment and disease process. Applicants must submit proof of completion of 40 or more hours of continuing education (CE) credits and multiple letters of recommendation from veterinarians, other VTSes or, with preference, a board-certified veterinary specialist.

If the application is accepted, applicants sit for the specialty examination, which may include demonstration of skill mastery, multiple choice questions, short-answer, and essay questions. After passing the validated examination, they are then required to recertify every 5^5 y, which involves submitting relevant CE, publishing, professional speaking, service to the veterinary profession, service to the academy, or re-taking the examination, all while maintaining their primary veterinary technician credential.[9,10]

CURRENT STATE OF DIVERSITY AMONG VETERINARY TECHNICIAN SPECIALISTS

When it comes to starting the conversation of increasing diversity specifically for VTSes, it is important to have foundational data to identify potential areas or groups that need attention. To collect these data, a 14-item electronic survey was sent to all the 16 NAVTA recognized veterinary technician specialty academies. The authors asked the academies to disseminate the survey to their member rosters via email, and the survey link was posted on the social media platform Facebook between January 20 and February 20, 2024. Survey items included demographic information, as well as asked for opinions on how to increase diversity and inclusion in the veterinary industry more broadly. Responses were quantitatively and qualitatively analyzed. The overall results align with other demographic studies published from other organizations and appear less diverse than the Bureau of Labor Statistics demographics.[1,2,11]

The number of respondents, 216, is statistically significant to reflect a 95% level of confidence in our sampling of the VTS community. Based on our collection of the total number of VTSes, which equated to 1534, the number of respondents provided us with a proportion of approximately 14% of all VTSes worldwide.

KEY POINTS NOTED IN THE VETERINARY TECHNICIAN SPECIALIST DATA

- Proportions of representation from the academies varied greatly.
- One VTS organization, the Academy of Veterinary Technicians in Diagnostic Imaging, had no respondents to the survey. There were 18 respondents that marked "2 or more academies", which also could correspond to the lack of representation from an academy as the respondents for this selection category were not asked to disclose which academies they belong to.
- There were no respondents that identified as Pacific Islander or Middle Eastern and Northern Africa. This could be due to the respondent sample size, or in fact a very small or complete lack of representation from these groups.
- A major lack of racial diversity is noted compared to the US racial demographics (**Figs. 1–12**).

REPRESENTATION MATTERS

The most recent US census data show 75.5% of the US population identifies as White, 19.1% Hispanic, 13.6% Black or African American, 6.3% Asian, 1.3% American Indian

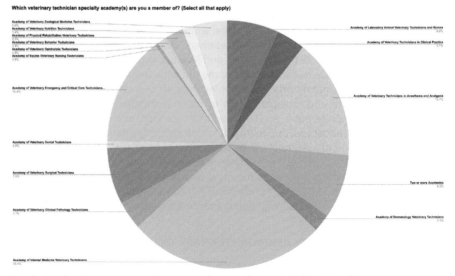

Fig. 1. Academies represented in survey data as shown in **Tables 1** and **2**.

How would you describe your gender?

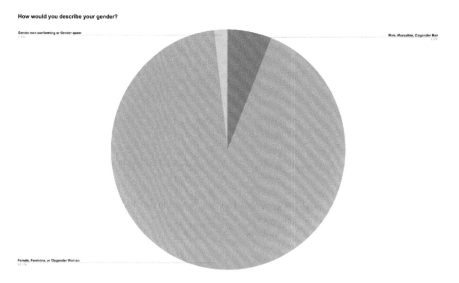

Female, Feminine, or Cisgender Woman	Male, Masculine, Cisgender Man	Gender Non-conforming or Gender queer
92.1%	6%	1.9%
This survey did not ask if respondents are transgendered out of respect for a person's self-described gender identity.		

Fig. 2. Gender demographics from survey respondents.

Age range demographics

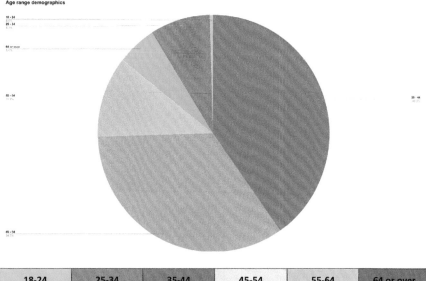

18-24	25-34	35-44	45-54	55-64	64 or over
0.5%	8.3%	40.3%	34.3%	11.1%	5.6%

Fig. 3. Age demographics from survey respondents.

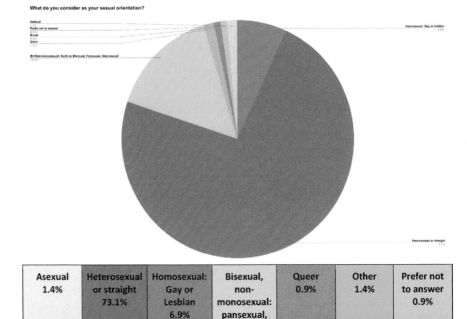

Fig. 4. Sexual orientation demographics from survey respondents.

Asexual 1.4%	Heterosexual or straight 73.1%	Homosexual: Gay or Lesbian 6.9%	Bisexual, non-monosexual: pansexual, omnisexual 15.3%	Queer 0.9%	Other 1.4%	Prefer not to answer 0.9%

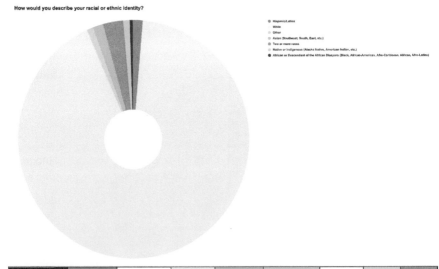

Fig. 5. Racial or ethnic demographics from survey respondents.

African or Descendant of the African Diaspora 0.5%	Hispanic/ Latinx 1.4%	Middle Eastern and Northern African 0%	White 92.1%	Asian 1.4%	Native or Indigenous 0.9%	Pacific Islander 0%	Other 0.9%	Two or more races 2.8%

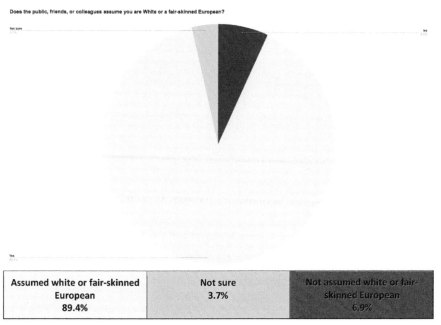

Fig. 6. Assumed white or fair-skinned European from all respondents.

and Alaska Native, and 0.3% Native Hawaiian and other Pacific Islander.[11] Compared to all other professions, in 2013, the veterinary industry was shown to be the most homogenous profession, with 91% to 92.4% White/non-Hispanic.[13,14] This homogeneity is seen with veterinary technicians, with 90% of NAVTA's 2022 demographic survey

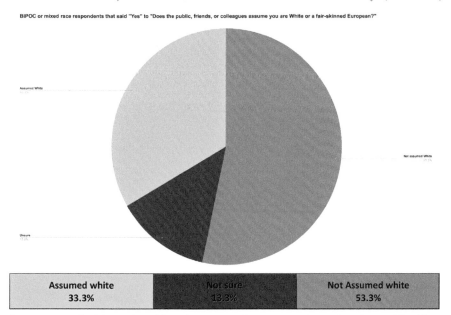

Fig. 7. Assumed white or fair-skinned European from respondents that do not identify as white.

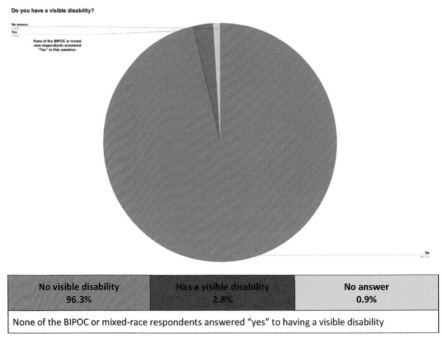

Fig. 8. Visible disability demographics from survey respondents.

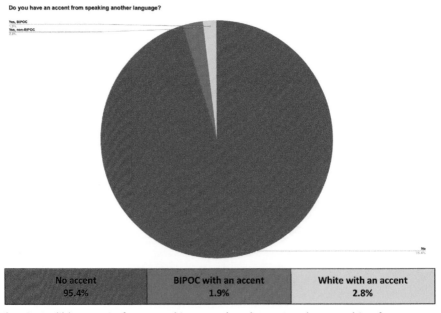

Fig. 9. Audible accent from speaking another language demographics from survey respondents.

Have you experienced any discrimination or bias within the veterinary industry based on any of your identities or visible differences?

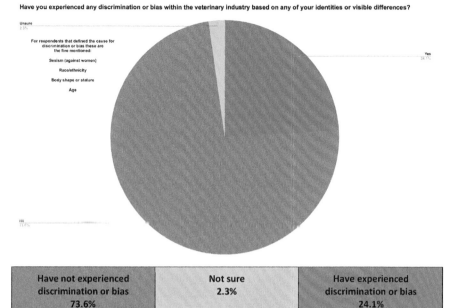

Have not experienced discrimination or bias 73.6%	Not sure 2.3%	Have experienced discrimination or bias 24.1%

Fig. 10. Demographics from survey respondents that have experienced discrimination or bias based off visible differences.

BIPOC respondents that have experienced discrimination or bias within the veterinary industry based on identity or visible differences?

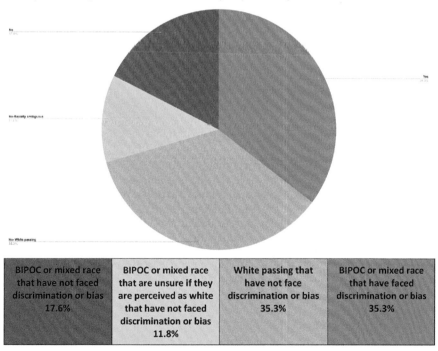

BIPOC or mixed race that have not faced discrimination or bias 17.6%	BIPOC or mixed race that are unsure if they are perceived as white that have not faced discrimination or bias 11.8%	White passing that have not face discrimination or bias 35.3%	BIPOC or mixed race that have faced discrimination or bias 35.3%

Fig. 11. Demographics from Black, Indigenous, and other People of Color (BIPOC) or mixed-race survey respondents that have experienced discrimination or bias based off visible differences.

Non-White passing or racially ambiguous people that have experienced discrimination or bias.

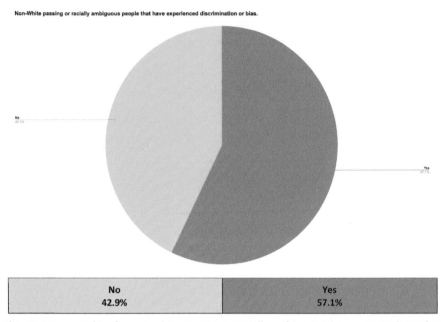

No	Yes
No 42.9%	**Yes** 57.1%

Fig. 12. Demographics for non-white passing or racially ambiguous survey respondents that have experienced discrimination or bias based on visible differences.

respondents identifying as Caucasian.[2] Out of just over 1500 veterinary technicians across the specialties, of the 216 that completed the VTS demographic survey, 92.1% identified as racially White. Lack of representation or visibility can create a perception that certain paths are not accessible or welcoming to individuals from diverse backgrounds, leading to limited career aspirations among minority veterinary professionals. Some communities may have limited exposure to veterinary services, leading to fewer individuals from these communities' pursuing careers in specialized veterinary fields.

*The 2022 NAVTA Demographic survey can be found here: http://bit.ly/3jY2WQG.

There is a concerning notion and growing hostility that DEIB initiatives are not significant, even divisive, and may detract from the focus on credentials and merit in the veterinary industry. This belief suggests that prioritizing DEIB efforts, particularly for BIPOC communities, somehow conflicts with the selection and training of highly qualified veterinary professionals. However, it is crucial to dispel these myths and emphasize the importance of DEIB in the field. Studies show that qualified candidates from underrepresented groups may not be applying to specialty programs due to a lack of opportunities in the pipeline, or worse that they "do not belong" based on generalized visual perceptions of those seen as representing a specialty. Somewhat dated research had previously highlighted gender segregation as a factor influencing decisions to apply for such programs, in this context residency programs, underscoring the need for targeted recruitment and pipeline development efforts for other underrepresented communities.[15–17] Other studies have shown that a more diverse pool of veterinary instructors is associated with increased interest in graduate programs, highlighting the significance of robust pipelines.[18,19]

Contrary to concerns that DEIB initiatives compromise the quality of trainees or medical practice, research in human medicine has demonstrated that including individuals from underrepresented backgrounds enhances patient care, improves

Table 1
Veterinary technician specialty academy representation

Academy	Total Members	Survey Respondents	Percent of Representation from Each Academy
Academy of Laboratory Animal Veterinary Technicians and Nurses	29	16	55%
Academy of Veterinary Technicians in Clinical Practice	59	12	20%
Academy of Veterinary Surgical Technicians	37	17	46%
Academy of Veterinary Dental Technicians	122	3	2%
Academy of Veterinary Nutrition Technicians	30	6	20%
Academy of Veterinary Technicians in Anesthesia and Analgesia	273	39	14%
Academy of Veterinary Zoologic Medicine Technicians	20	10	50%
Academy of Physical Rehabilitation Veterinary Technicians	16	6	38%
Academy of Veterinary Clinical Pathology Technicians	12	8	67%
Academy of Internal Medicine Veterinary Technicians	228	67	29%
Academy of Veterinary Emergency and Critical Care Technicians and Nurses	587	40	7%
Academy of Veterinary Equine Nursing Technicians	28	1	3%
Academy of Veterinary Behavior Technicians	29	2	7%
Academy of Dermatology Veterinary Technicians	15	5	33%
Academy of Veterinary Technicians in Diagnostic Imaging	21	0	0%
Academy of Veterinary Ophthalmic Technicians	28	2	7%
Two or more Academies	Unknown	18	NA
Totals	1534	216	14% overall representation

Data for this chart were collected by the authors asking the individual Academies for their member numbers. This was compared to the 2023 Committee of Veterinary Technicians Specialties member numbers submitted to the CVTS during their annual review process. Total respondent numbers from the survey were then added to create the table.

Table 2
Race and ethnicity categories

US Federal Government's Race and Ethnicity Categories 1997.	US Federal Government's Race and Ethnicity Categories 2024. (Adopted March 28th, 2024) now Allowed to Mark all that Apply.	Race and Ethnicity Categories Used in VTS® Survey Data Collection.
Black or African American A person having origins in any of the black racial groups of Africa.	Black or African American African American, Jamaican, Haitian, Nigerian, Ethiopian, Somali, etc.	African or Descendant of the African Diaspora Black, African American, Afro-Caribbean, African, Afro-Latinx
White A person having origins in any of the original peoples of Europe, the Middle East, or North Africa.	White English, German, Irish, Italian, Polish, Scottish, etc.	White
	Middle Eastern or North African Lebanese, Iranian, Egyptian, Syrian, Iraqi, Israeli, etc.	Middle Eastern and Northern African Algerian, Egyptian, Iranian, Moroccan, Palestinian, Saudi Arabian, Israeli, etc.
American Indian or Alaska Native A person having origins in any of the original peoples of North and South America (including Central America), and who maintains tribal affiliation or community attachment.	American Indian or Alaska Native Navajo Nation, Blackfeet Tribe of the Blackfeet Indian Reservation of Montana, Native Village of Barrow Inupiat Traditional Government, Nome Eskimo Community, Aztec, Maya, etc.	Native or Indigenous Alaska Native, Native American, Indigenous Latin American or mix.
Asian A person having origins in any of the original peoples of the Far East, Southeast Asia, or the Indian subcontinent, including, for example, Cambodia, China, India, Japan, Korea, Malaysia, Pakistan, the Philippine Islands, Thailand, and Vietnam.	Asian Chinese, Asian Indian, Filipino, Vietnamese, Korean, Japanese, etc.	Asian Southeast, South, East, etc.
Native Hawaiian or Other Pacific Islander A person having origins in any of the original peoples of Hawaii, Guam, Samoa, or other Pacific Islands.	Native Hawaiian or Other Pacific Islander Native Hawaiian, Samoan, Chamorro, Tongan, Fijian, Marshallese, etc.)	Pacific Islanders Polynesian, Melanesian, Micronesian, Native Hawaiian, etc.
*Ethnicity qualifier after checking a race category: Hispanic or Latino A person of Cuban, Mexican, Puerto Rican, Cuban, South or Central American, or other Spanish culture or origin, regardless of race.	Hispanic of Latino Mexican, Puerto Rican, Salvadoran, Cuban, Dominican, Guatemalan, etc.	Two or more races
		Other: with option to fill in space

The United States of America's 1997 and 2024 Office of Information and Regulatory Affairs, Office of Management and Budget, and Executive Office of the Pres-healthcare quality, and fosters diverse perspectives that drive innovation in medical research.[20,21]

Challenges Faced by Black, Indigenous, and Other People of Color in Pursuing Their Veterinary Technician Specialty

Pursuing a career in veterinary medicine is an admirable and rewarding career path. It is no less rewarding for a CrVT advancing within the profession as a VTS in 1 of the 28 recognized specialties than a veterinarian finishing a residency program and passing their specialty board examination. However, the journey to becoming a CrVT and/or VTS for BIPOC is filled with underestimated challenges stemming from long-standing systemic socio-economic issues, lack of representation, and early mentorship. Other factors, such as the limited exposure to educational and professional pathways may also play a factor. For example, both authors for this article were unaware of veterinary technology, let alone specialization during high school. The underrepresentation of BIPOC within the profession at large and within the veterinary technician specialties warrants open dialogue that can lead to an actionable pathway to diversifying the VTS pipeline. Here, we briefly discuss common themes that contribute to a dysfunctional pipeline.

Financial Challenges and Barriers to Entry to the Veterinary Technician Specialist Pathway

The cost of the VTS application process can vary based on academy requirements, examination methods, and fees. For the currently approved academies, an applicant must complete a specific number of specialty-specific clinical hours and additional CE hours to fulfill the initial application process. The general cost of obtaining a VTS can present a financial barrier for any applicant. According to the 2022 NAVTA demographic survey, the average hourly rate of a CrVT in the US is $26.50, with a median rate of $23 per hour with a median average salary of $45,700.[2] Though increased from previous surveys, this wage, factored with financial obligations, cost of living, student debt, and personal debt, limits the available financial resources for any interested applicant and puts the feasibility of pursuing additional advancement lower on the list of priorities. This is especially true for the BIPOC applicants who may have financial constraints from historically systemic challenges, family obligations including multigeneration households, which are more prevalent in BIPOC communities, lack of parental and other family support, and lack of established generational wealth and security.[22] BIPOC and other underrepresented groups may not always be able to prioritize taking additional steps to elevate their career beyond those that will only help alleviate other responsibilities. Financial and family obligations, among other factors, can steer them to more lucrative occupations and help quell more immediate concerns.

In addition, completing specialty-specific CE often requires an applicant to incur additional financial commitments to achieve a specialty. From registering for applicable CE to attending specialty meetings and conferences, obtaining the pre-application requirements can be costly. The financial commitment to attend a conference will require registration fees, travel, and hotel accommodation. Attending more than 1 conference is often necessary for some applicants to obtain the required CE, increasing the financial burden. Some academies require in-person CE instead of virtual options. Annually, the cost of attending conferences has consistently risen, making the financial path to success daunting for applicants. The financial commitment cannot be underscored as a roadblock to diversifying the VTS pipeline. Over the past several years, CrVTs have seen improvements in compensation and other benefits. Employers offering to pay for full or partial CE provide a reprieve and mutual opportunity. Communities that are historically not as disadvantaged as BIPOC communities can also suffer from economic stress, but it should be noted they also statistically do not have the same or as many hurdles in access to various resources.[23–25]

Awareness, Advocacy, and Competency

As veterinary medicine navigates the lack of diversity, CrVTs and VTSes must engage in dialogue focusing on DEIB and strategies to increase diversity within the specialties. To the authors' knowledge, there has been limited (but increasing) discussion in the space of DEIB. NAVTA reports that approximately 90% of members who responded to their 2022 demographic survey are White or Caucasian. The result of the VTS demographic survey aligns with NAVTA's survey of CrVTs and provides a foundation for continued discussion. With several other issues at the forefront of the profession, including defining national credentialing guidelines, title and title protection, and technician utilization, adding DEIB can be regarded as a daunting task, yet vital to the profession's progress. With over 90% of CrVTs and the VTS community homogeneously White, educating the profession on the importance of DEIB as part of strategic planning may clear the pathway for change. Diversity benefits organizations by providing alternate perspectives and experiences, increasing revenue streams, and providing long-term solutions and innovations. The CVTS in their most updated policies and procedures includes a recommendation to academies that states:

"Include a Diversity, Equity, and Inclusion statement that the VTSA believes in and upholds. Veterinary Technician Specialty Academies may use verbiage at their discretion; however, suggested wording is as follows: The XXXXX (VTSA) is committed to diversity and inclusion in all aspects of the profession so that we can best serve our members and the animals in their care. We are committed to actively promoting and maintaining diversity and inclusion in our membership, leadership, and organization, and educating our members regarding the value of diversity and inclusion. We also embrace a zero-tolerance policy of all forms of DEI harassment which may result in expulsion from the VTSA and/or banning from VTSA events. This commitment embraces the value of our members' varied backgrounds, including but not limited to race; ethnicity; physical and mental abilities; gender; sexual orientation; gender identity or expression; parental, marital, or pregnancy status; religious or political beliefs; military or veteran status; and geographic, socioeconomic, and educational backgrounds."[9]

While the definition of "cultural competence" evolves, its essence is the understanding and respect of cultures and perspectives that are different from one's own.[26] As a demographically homogeneous profession, there is a need for awareness of the lack of diversity and its impact on the profession and patient care. The NAVTA created a DEIB committee to promote the importance of DEIB for veterinary technicians. This committee is a step toward increasing awareness, implementing measures to understand the significance of DEIB, and providing its members with resources, training, and education. These strategies can increase awareness and improve traction toward cultural competence and cultural intelligence of the organization and its members. However, while well-indented, such committees and statements as seen earlier are often hollow with little action made to ensure the charge of the committee or statements are achieved or enforced.

Mentorship and Early Professional Development and Support

It has been widely recognized that successful mentorship programs provide a positive mutual outcome for the mentee and mentor. Mentorship is defined as a relationship that helps to build and support the professional career of a less experienced individual by imparting knowledge, time, and experience to maximize a successful career. The 2023 AAHA Mentoring Guidelines describe various mentorship models that can be leveraged to impart knowledge, transition through different stages of one's career, build a network, and foster lifelong professional relationships.

*The AAHA Mentoring Guidelines can be found here: https://www.aaha.org/aaha-guidelines/2023-aaha-mentoring-guidelines/home/

The VTS academies also utilize various mentorship modules geared toward individuals who have already decided to become specialists. However, diversifying the VTS pipeline would require initiatives before this decision is made, as well as a more serious investigation into attracting BIPOC to veterinary technology. The best mentorship comes from someone who can relate to a mentee's lived experience, understands the challenges they may have gone through, and communicates in a similar way (verbally or non-verbally) to build personal connection. Mentorship by a BIPOC individual to another BIPOC individual is ideal but given the data and not wanting to overburden the few BIPOC VTSes that exist can make this challenging.

Greenhill and colleagues discuss multiple factors that impact the career decisions of young Black and Hispanic students. For many, career aspirations, even at a young age, are influenced by the occupations that surround them. Early career interventions and exposure to CrVTs and the VTS career pathway should be considered. This can be accomplished through community outreach programs, collaboration with local education programs, and career days to introduce and expose individuals to various career options, including pursuing a veterinary technician specialty.

An introspective reflection is also needed. The VTS demographic survey serves as a way to continue the dialogue on the current state of this group of veterinary professionals. With less than 10% of respondents identifying as not White, taking on this challenge within the VTS pipeline is no less daunting than that for veterinarians.

CrVTs and the VTS academies can introspectively promote education and the importance of diversity to their members. Improving education and understanding the long-standing systemic challenges faced by underrepresented groups within the profession can also help identify allies to further the importance of diversity. Initiatives to improve cultural competency and cultural intelligence are important measures that are largely overlooked.

Identifying as an ally is one way anyone can help improve diversity. An ally is any individual who understands that there are members of groups besides the one they identify with and acknowledges with humility that marginalized and underrepresented communities face oppression and inequities that are deeply rooted in society. They strive to gain knowledge of the challenges faced by underrepresented groups and support actions to make positive change.

SUMMARY

While challenges exist, there are opportunities for diversifying specialization for veterinary technicians. Addressing these opportunities requires a multi-faceted approach that involves collaboration among educational institutions, professional organizations, policymakers, and industry stakeholders.

Fostering diversity and inclusivity in the veterinary industry, particularly in specialization, is critical for promoting equity, improving patient care, and driving innovation.

DISCLOSURE

The authors have nothing to disclose.

REFERENCES

1. Paschal-Bennett L. Championing diversity in veterinary medicine. Today's Veterinary Business. 2023. Available at: https://todaysveterinarybusiness.com/diversity-viewpoints-1223/. Accessed April 1, 2024.
2. Friesen M. NAVTA survey reveals veterinary technician pay and education have increased, but burnout, debt are still issues. NAVTA. 2023. Available at: https://navta.net/news/navta-survey-reveals-veterinary-technician-pay-and-education-have-increased-but-burnout-debt-are-still-issues-2/.
3. Veterinary technologists and technicians | Data USA. datausa.io. Accessed April 4, 2024. Available at: https://datausa.io/profile/soc/veterinary-technologists-and-technicians#:~:text=In%202021%2C%2082.1%25%20of%20the.
4. Daniel A. Creating a path to diversity in the veterinary profession. today's veterinary practice. 2021. Available at: https://www.researchgate.net/profile/Annie-Daniel/publication/351346762_Creating_a_Path_to_Diversity_in_the_Veterinary_Profession/links/6092882ca6fdccaebd096dd6/Creating-a-Path-to-Diversity-in-the-Veterinary-Profession.pdf. Accessed February 2, 2024.
5. Odunayo & Ng, (2021) in Valuing Diversity in the Team, Veterinary Clinics of North America: Small Animal Practice.
6. How diversity, equity, and inclusion (DE&I) matter | McKinsey. Available at: www.mckinsey.com. https://www.mckinsey.com/featured-insights/diversity-and-inclusion/diversity-wins-how-inclusion-matters#/.
7. Campaign highlights importance of vet nurses/techs. NAVC. 2023. Available at: https://navc.com/campaign-highlights-importance-of-vet-nurses-techs/. Accessed April 4, 2024.
8. Veterinary technicians and veterinary assistants | American Veterinary Medical Association. Available at: www.avma.org. Accessed April 4, 2024.
9. Veterinary technician specialties. NAVTA. Available at: https://navta.net/veterinary-technician-specialties/.
10. Cital S. An Established Solution for a Rising Problem. AAHA. Published October 2022. Accessed April 24, 3AD. https://www.aaha.org/publications/trends-magazine/trends-articles/2022/october-2022/gs-vts/
11. Bureau UC. 2020 census illuminates racial and ethnic composition of the country. Census.gov. Available at: https://www.census.gov/library/stories/2021/08/improved-race-ethnicity-measures-reveal-united-states-population-much-more-multiracial.html#:~:text=The2020CensusshowsFigures.
12. Federal register. Available at: https://www.federalregister.gov/documents/2024/03/29/2024-06469/revisions-to-ombs-statistical-policy-directive-no-15-standards-for-maintaining-collecting-and. Accessed April 4, 2024.
13. The Whitest Jobs. Zippia. 2021. Available at: https://www.zippia.com/advice/the-whitest-jobs/.
14. Thompson D. The Atlantic. 2013. Available at: https://www.theatlantic.com/business/archive/2013/11/the-33-whitest-jobs-in-america/281180/.
15. Gonzalez LM, Stampley AR, Marcellin-Little DJ, et al. Respondents to an American College of Veterinary Surgeons diplomate survey support the promotion of diversity, equity, and inclusion initiatives. J Am Vet Med Assoc 2023;261(12):1847–52.

16. Moore S, Fielding J, MacDermott C. Barriers to female career progression in medicine. Future Healthcare Journal 2017;4(Suppl 2):s28.
17. Tsugawa Y, Jena AB, Figueroa JF, et al. Comparison of hospital mortality and re-admission rates for medicare patients treated by male vs female physicians. JAMA Intern Med 2017;177(2):206.
18. Greenhill L, Davis K, Lowrie P, et al. Navigating diversity and inclusion in veterinary medicine. Purdue University. 2020. Available at: https://www.press.purdue.edu/9781612496689/.
19. Elce Y. The mentor-mentee relationship, addressing challenges in veterinary medicine together. Vet Clin Small Anim Pract 2021;51(5):1099–109. https://doi.org/10.1016/j.cvsm.2021.04.023.
20. Gomez LE, Bernet P. Diversity improves performance and outcomes. J Natl Med Assoc 2019;111(4):383–92.
21. Zephyrin L, Rodriguez J, Rosenbaum S. The Case for Diversity in the Health Professions Remains Powerful. www.commonwealthfund.org. Published July 20, 2023. Available at: https://www.commonwealthfund.org/blog/2023/case-diversity-health-professions-remains-powerful.
22. Cohn D, Passel JS. A record 64 million Americans live in multigenerational households. Pew Research Center. 2018. Available at: https://www.pewresearch.org/short-reads/2018/04/05/a-record-64-million-americans-live-in-multigenerational-households/.
23. Weller C. African Americans face systematic obstacles to getting good jobs. Center for American Progress. 2019. Available at: https://www.americanprogress.org/article/african-americans-face-systematic-obstacles-getting-good-jobs/.
24. APA. "Ethnic and racial minorities & socioeconomic status." American Psychological Association. 2017. Available at: www.apa.org/pi/ses/resources/publications/minorities.
25. Pager D, Bonikowski B, Western B. Discrimination in a low-wage labor market. Am Socio Rev 2009;74(5):777–99.
26. Georgetown University. Definitions of cultural competence. Georgetown.edu. 2019. Available at: https://nccc.georgetown.edu/curricula/culturalcompetence.html.

UNITED STATES POSTAL SERVICE® Statement of Ownership, Management, and Circulation (All Periodicals Publications Except Requester Publications)

1. Publication Title VETERINARY CLINICS OF NORTH AMERICA: SMALL ANIMAL PRACTICE	**2. Publication Number** 003 – 150	**3. Filing Date** 5/18/2024
4. Issue Frequency JAN, MAR, MAY, JUL, SEP, NOV	**5. Number of Issues Published Annually** 6	**6. Annual Subscription Price** $391.00

7. Complete Mailing Address of Known Office of Publication *(Not printer)* *(Street, city, county, state, and ZIP+4®)*
ELSEVIER INC.
230 Park Avenue, Suite 800
New York, NY 10169

Contact Person: Malathi Samayan
Telephone *(Include area code)*: 98I-44-4299-4507

8. Complete Mailing Address of Headquarters or General Business Office of Publisher *(Not printer)*
ELSEVIER INC.
230 Park Avenue, Suite 800
New York, NY 10169

9. Full Names and Complete Mailing Addresses of Publisher, Editor, and Managing Editor *(Do not leave blank)*

Publisher *(Name and complete mailing address)*
Dolores Meloni, ELSEVIER INC.
1600 JOHN F KENNEDY BLVD. SUITE 1600
PHILADELPHIA, PA 19103-2899

Editor *(Name and complete mailing address)*
STACY EASTMAN, ELSEVIER INC.
1600 JOHN F KENNEDY BLVD. SUITE 1600
PHILADELPHIA, PA 19103-2899

Managing Editor *(Name and complete mailing address)*
PATRICK MANLEY, ELSEVIER INC.
1600 JOHN F KENNEDY BLVD. SUITE 1600
PHILADELPHIA, PA 19103-2899

10. Owner *(Do not leave blank. If the publication is owned by a corporation, give the name and address of the corporation immediately followed by the names and addresses of all stockholders owning or holding 1 percent or more of the total amount of stock. If not owned by a corporation, give the names and addresses of the individual owners. If owned by a partnership or other unincorporated firm, give its name and address as well as those of each individual owner. If the publication is published by a nonprofit organization, give its name and address.)*

Full Name	Complete Mailing Address
WHOLLY OWNED SUBSIDIARY OF REED/ELSEVIER, US HOLDINGS	1600 JOHN F KENNEDY BLVD. SUITE 160C PHILADELPHIA, PA 19103-2899

11. Known Bondholders, Mortgagees, and Other Security Holders Owning or Holding 1 Percent or More of Total Amount of Bonds, Mortgages, or Other Securities. If none, check box. ☑ None

Full Name	Complete Mailing Address
N/A	

12. Tax Status *(For completion by nonprofit organizations authorized to mail at nonprofit rates)* *(Check one)*
The purpose, function, and nonprofit status of this organization and the exempt status for federal income tax purposes:
☒ Has Not Changed During Preceding 12 Months
☐ Has Changed During Preceding 12 Months *(Publisher must submit explanation of change with this statement)*

PS Form **3526**, July 2014 [Page 1 of 4 (see instructions page 4)]   PSN: 7530-01-000-9931   PRIVACY NOTICE: See our privacy policy on www.usps.com.

---

13. Publication Title VETERINARY CLINICS OF NORTH AMERICA: SMALL ANIMAL PRACTICE	**14. Issue Date for Circulation Data Below** JULY 2024

15. Extent and Nature of Circulation		Average No. Copies Each Issue During Preceding 12 Months	No. Copies of Single Issue Published Nearest to Filing Date
a. Total Number of Copies *(Net press run)*		368	343
b. Paid Circulation *(By Mail and Outside the Mail)*	(1) Mailed Outside-County Paid Subscriptions Stated on PS Form 3541 *(Include paid distribution above nominal rate, advertiser's proof copies, and exchange copies)*	237	212
	(2) Mailed In-County Paid Subscriptions Stated on PS Form 3541 *(Include paid distribution above nominal rate, advertiser's proof copies, and exchange copies)*	0	0
	(3) Paid Distribution Outside the Mails Including Sales Through Dealers and Carriers, Street Vendors, Counter Sales, and Other Paid Distribution Outside USPS®	118	119
	(4) Paid Distribution by Other Classes of Mail Through the USPS *(e.g., First-Class Mail®)*	7	6
c. Total Paid Distribution *(Sum of 15b (1), (2), (3), and (4))*	▲	362	337
d. Free or Nominal Rate Distribution *(By Mail and Outside the Mail)*	(1) Free or Nominal Rate Outside-County Copies included on PS Form 3541	5	5
	(2) Free or Nominal Rate In-County Copies Included on PS Form 3541	0	0
	(3) Free or Nominal Rate Copies Mailed at Other Classes Through the USPS *(e.g., First-Class Mail)*	0	0
	(4) Free or Nominal Rate Distribution Outside the Mail *(Carriers or other means)*	1	1
e. Total Free or Nominal Rate Distribution *(Sum of 15d (1), (2), (3) and (4))*	▲	6	6
f. Total Distribution *(Sum of 15c and 15e)*	▲	368	343
g. Copies not Distributed *(See Instructions to Publishers #4 (page #3))*	▲	0	0
h. Total *(Sum of 15f and g)*		368	343
i. Percent Paid *(15c divided by 15f times 100)*	▲	98.37%	98.25%

* If you are claiming electronic copies, go to line 16 on page 3. If you are not claiming electronic copies, skip to line 17 on page 3.

PS Form **3526**, July 2014 (Page 2 of 4)

16. Electronic Copy Circulation		Average No. Copies Each Issue During Preceding 12 Months	No. Copies of Single Issue Published Nearest to Filing Date
a. Paid Electronic Copies	▲		
b. Total Paid Print Copies (Line 15c) + Paid Electronic Copies (Line 16a)	▲		
c. Total Print Distribution (Line 15f) + Paid Electronic Copies (Line 16a)	▲		
d. Percent Paid (Both Print & Electronic Copies) (16b divided by 16c × 100)	▲		

☒ I certify that 50% of all my distributed copies (electronic and print) are paid above a nominal price.

17. Publication of Statement of Ownership
☒ If the publication is a general publication, publication of this statement is required. Will be printed in the NOVEMBER 2024 issue of this publication.   ☐ Publication not required.

18. Signature and Title of Editor, Publisher, Business Manager, or Owner
Malathi Samayan — Malathi Samayan - Distribution Controller   Date 9/18/2024

I certify that all information furnished on this form is true and complete. I understand that anyone who furnishes false or misleading information on this form or who omits material or information requested on the form may be subject to criminal sanctions (including fines and imprisonment) and/or civil sanctions (including civil penalties).

PS Form **3526**, July 2014 (Page 3 of 4)   PRIVACY NOTICE: See our privacy policy on www.usps.com

Printed and bound by CPI Group (UK) Ltd, Croydon, CR0 4YY

08/05/2025

01864752-0006